Introduction

Welcome to ***"110+ Low-Fiber Recipes for Diverticulitis: Gentle and Delicious Meals."*** This book is thoughtfully designed to support individuals dealing with diverticulitis by providing a comprehensive collection of low-fiber recipes that are as nourishing as they are delectable. Understanding the dietary needs of those managing this condition, we have created this resource to help you enjoy food without compromising your health.

Diverticulitis is a condition that involves the inflammation or infection of diverticula—small pouches that can form in the walls of the colon. During flare-ups, a low-fiber diet is often recommended to minimize irritation and allow the digestive system to heal. This cookbook aims to simplify the process of adhering to a low-fiber diet by offering a diverse range of recipes that are easy to prepare, gentle on the stomach, and packed with flavor.

In this book, you will find over 110 recipes specifically tailored to meet the dietary requirements of individuals with diverticulitis. From breakfast to dinner, snacks to desserts, each recipe is carefully crafted to provide maximum nutrition while being gentle on your digestive system. You will discover a variety of dishes that cater to different tastes and dietary preferences, ensuring that you can enjoy satisfying meals without the worry of aggravating your condition.

We begin with an informative introduction to diverticulitis, explaining the role of a low-fiber diet in managing symptoms and promoting recovery. Understanding the importance of ingredient selection and cooking methods is crucial, and we offer practical tips and guidelines to help you make informed decisions in your kitchen. Whether you are new to cooking or a seasoned chef, you will find these recipes straightforward and accessible, designed to make your culinary experience both enjoyable and healthful.

Each recipe in this book is created with easily digestible ingredients and includes step-by-step instructions to ensure success. We also provide nutritional information and tips for adapting recipes to suit your individual needs. Our goal is to make mealtime a positive and stress-free experience, helping you maintain a balanced diet that supports your health journey.

"110+ Low-Fiber Recipes for Diverticulitis" is more than just a cookbook; it is a tool to empower you in your daily life. By incorporating these gentle and delicious meals into your diet, you can manage your diverticulitis symptoms effectively while still enjoying the pleasures of eating.

We invite you to explore these recipes, embrace the process of cooking, and discover how a thoughtful, low-fiber diet can enhance your well-being. Here's to your health, happiness, and the comforting meals that lie ahead.

1. Scrambled Eggs

Ingredients:
- 3 eggs
- 1 tbsp butter or oil
- 2 tbsp milk or cream (optional)
- Salt and pepper to taste

Instructions:

1. Crack the eggs into a bowl and beat them lightly with a fork or whisk until blended. Add the milk/cream if using and season with salt and pepper.

2. Heat a non-stick skillet over medium heat and melt the butter or heat the oil.

3. Pour the egg mixture into the hot pan. As the eggs start to set around the edges, use a spatula to gently push the cooked eggs towards the center, tilting the pan to allow the uncooked egg to flow to the edges.

4. Continue this gentle folding and stirring motion until the eggs are mostly set but still look a bit moist, about 2-3 minutes total.

5. Remove from heat and continue folding/stirring for another 30 seconds as the eggs will continue to cook off the heat.

6. Serve the scrambled eggs immediately, while hot. Adjust seasoning as needed.

Tips:
- For creamier scrambled eggs, use a bit more milk/cream.

- Don't overcook the eggs - they should still look a bit soft and moist when removed from the heat.

- Experiment with add-ins like cheese, herbs, or diced veggies.

2. Mashed Potatoes

Ingredients:
- 3 lbs Russet or Yukon Gold potatoes, peeled and cut into 1-inch chunks
- 1 cup milk, warmed
- 4 tbsp unsalted butter, softened
- 1 tsp salt
- 1/4 tsp black pepper

Instructions:

1. Place the potato chunks in a large pot and cover with cold water by 1 inch. Bring to a boil over high heat.

2. Once boiling, reduce heat to medium-low and simmer for 15-20 minutes, until the potatoes are very tender when pierced with a fork.

3. Drain the potatoes in a colander and return them to the hot pot for 1 minute to evaporate any excess moisture.

4. Add the warm milk, butter, salt, and pepper. Mash the potatoes with a potato masher or ricer until smooth and creamy.

5. Taste and adjust seasoning as needed, adding more salt, pepper, butter or milk to reach your desired consistency and flavor.

6. Serve the mashed potatoes hot, garnished with extra butter, chives, or other toppings if desired.

Tips:
- For extra creamy potatoes, use a ricer or food mill instead of a masher.

- Add roasted garlic, cheese, or herbs to customize the flavor.

- Use a combination of potatoes for different textures.

- Don't overmix the potatoes or they can become gummy.

3. Plain White Rice

Ingredients:
- 1 cup long-grain white rice (such as basmati or jasmine)
- 1 1/2 cups water
- 1/4 tsp salt (optional)

Instructions:

1. Rinse the rice: Place the rice in a fine mesh strainer and rinse it under cool running water, stirring the rice with your hand, until the water runs clear. This helps remove excess starch.

2. Combine the rice, water, and salt (if using) in a medium saucepan. Bring to a boil over high heat.

3. Once boiling, cover the pot with a tight-fitting lid and reduce the heat to the lowest setting. Simmer for 15-18 minutes, without lifting the lid.

4. After 15-18 minutes, remove the pot from the heat and let it sit, covered, for an additional 5-10 minutes. This allows the rice to finish steaming and become perfectly tender.

5. Fluff the rice with a fork before serving.

Tips:
- Use a 1:1.5 rice to water ratio for perfectly cooked rice.

- For extra flavor, substitute chicken or vegetable broth for the water.

- Add a pat of butter or drizzle of olive oil after cooking for extra richness.

- Experiment with different types of rice - brown, wild, or basmati all work well.

4. Boiled Chicken Breast

Ingredients:
- 4 boneless, skinless chicken breasts
- 4 cups chicken broth or water
- 1 tsp salt
- 1/2 tsp black pepper

Instructions:

1. Place the chicken breasts in a large pot and cover with the chicken broth or water. Add the salt and pepper.

2. Bring the liquid to a boil over high heat. Once boiling, reduce the heat to low, cover the pot with a lid, and simmer for 12-15 minutes, or until the chicken is cooked through.

3. Use a meat thermometer to check that the internal temperature of the chicken reaches 165°F. The chicken should be opaque throughout and the juices should run clear when pierced.

4. Carefully remove the cooked chicken breasts from the pot using tongs or a slotted spoon.

5. Allow the chicken to rest for 5 minutes before slicing or shredding. This allows the juices to redistribute throughout the meat.

6. Serve the boiled chicken breasts warm, or refrigerate and use in salads, sandwiches, or other recipes.

Tips:
- For extra flavor, add aromatics like onion, garlic, herbs, or lemon to the poaching liquid.

- Adjust the cooking time based on the size of your chicken breasts. Thicker pieces may need an extra 2-3 minutes.

- Reserve the poaching liquid to use as a base for soups or sauces.

- Shred or dice the cooked chicken for easy meal prep.

5. Poached Eggs

Ingredients:
- 4 fresh eggs
- 2 cups water
- 1 tbsp white vinegar
- 1/4 tsp salt

Instructions:

1. Fill a medium saucepan with 2 cups of water and bring it to a gentle simmer over medium heat. Add the white vinegar and salt.

2. Crack each egg individually into a small ramekin or cup. This will make it easier to gently slide the egg into the simmering water.

3. Carefully slide the eggs, one at a time, into the simmering water. Poach for 4-5 minutes for a soft, runny yolk, or 5-6 minutes for a more set yolk.

4. Use a slotted spoon to gently remove the poached eggs from the water, allowing any excess water to drain off.

5. Serve the poached eggs immediately, on top of toast, English muffins, or as part of a larger breakfast dish.

Tips:
- Use the freshest eggs possible for best results. Older eggs tend to spread out more in the water.

- Adding vinegar to the poaching water helps the eggs hold their shape.

- Adjust the cooking time to your desired doneness of the yolk.

- For perfectly round poached eggs, you can use egg poaching cups or rings in the simmering water.

- Top the poached eggs with hollandaise sauce, avocado, or other favorite toppings.

6. White Bread Toast

Ingredients:
- 4 slices of white sandwich bread
- Butter or margarine (optional)

Instructions:

1. Place the slices of white bread into a toaster or toaster oven.

2. Toast the bread on a medium to medium-high setting until it reaches your desired level of doneness, usually 2-3 minutes.

3. Keep a close eye on the toast to prevent it from burning. The bread should be golden brown in color.

4. Once the toast is ready, remove it from the toaster and place it on a plate or cutting board.

5. If desired, spread a thin layer of butter or margarine over the hot toast.

6. Serve the white bread toast immediately, while it's still warm and crispy.

Tips:
- Use fresh, high-quality white sandwich bread for the best results.

- Adjust the toaster setting based on your personal preference for crispness.

- Try different types of bread, such as whole wheat or sourdough, for variety.

- Top the toast with your favorite toppings, such as jam, honey, peanut butter, or avocado.

- For extra flavor, try rubbing a cut garlic clove over the hot toast.

7. Chicken Broth

Ingredients:
- 3-4 lbs chicken bones and/or carcass (from a roasted chicken)
- 1 onion, roughly chopped
- 2 carrots, roughly chopped
- 2 celery stalks, roughly chopped
- 3 garlic cloves, peeled
- 1 bay leaf
- 1 tsp whole peppercorns
- 1 tsp salt (or to taste)
- 8 cups cold water

Instructions:

1. Place the chicken bones, onion, carrots, celery, garlic, bay leaf, and peppercorns in a large stockpot or Dutch oven. Pour in the cold water and add the salt.

2. Bring the mixture to a boil over high heat. Once boiling, reduce the heat to low, cover the pot with a lid, and let the broth simmer for 2-3 hours, skimming any foam or fat that rises to the surface.

3. After simmering, remove the pot from the heat and let it cool slightly. Strain the broth through a fine-mesh sieve, discarding the solids.

4. Allow the broth to cool completely, then transfer it to airtight containers or jars. Refrigerate for up to 1 week or freeze for up to 3 months.

Tips:
- Use a combination of chicken bones, wings, and/or a leftover roasted chicken carcass for the best flavor.
- Roast the chicken bones and vegetables first for a deeper, richer broth.

- Add other herbs and spices like thyme, parsley, or ginger for extra flavor.

- Use the broth in soups, stews, rice dishes, or simply enjoy it on its own.

- Freeze the broth in ice cube trays for easy portioning.

8. Plain Pasta

Ingredients:
- 8 oz (225g) dry pasta (such as spaghetti, penne, or fusilli)
- 4 cups (1 liter) water
- 1 tsp salt

Instructions:

1. Bring a large pot of water to a rapid boil over high heat. Add the salt to the water.

2. Once the water is boiling, add the dry pasta. Stir gently to prevent the pasta from sticking together.

3. Cook the pasta according to the package instructions, usually 8-12 minutes for most dried pasta varieties. Stir occasionally during cooking.

4. To test for doneness, take a piece of pasta out of the water and taste it. It should be tender but still have a slight bite (al dente).

5. Once the pasta is cooked to your desired texture, drain it through a colander or fine mesh strainer. Be sure to drain the pasta well, shaking the colander to remove any excess water.

6. Serve the plain cooked pasta immediately, or toss it with your desired sauce, vegetables, or other ingredients.

Tips:
- Use a large pot with plenty of water to allow the pasta to cook evenly without sticking.

- Salt the cooking water generously to season the pasta.

- Don't rinse the cooked pasta, as this will wash away the starch that helps the sauce cling to the noodles.

- For extra flavor, cook the pasta in chicken or vegetable broth instead of water.

- Toss the hot, drained pasta with a bit of olive oil or butter to prevent it from sticking together

9. Baked Fish

Ingredients:
- 4 (6 oz) fish fillets (such as tilapia, cod, or salmon)
- 2 tbsp olive oil or melted butter
- 1 tsp lemon juice
- 1 tsp dried parsley (or 1 tbsp fresh chopped parsley)
- 1/2 tsp salt
- 1/4 tsp black pepper

Instructions:

1. Preheat your oven to 400°F (200°C).

2. Pat the fish fillets dry with paper towels and place them in a baking dish or on a rimmed baking sheet lined with parchment paper.

3. In a small bowl, mix together the olive oil or melted butter, lemon juice, parsley, salt, and pepper.

4. Brush or spoon the seasoned oil mixture over the top of the fish fillets, making sure to evenly coat them.

5. Bake the fish in the preheated oven for 12-15 minutes, or until the fish flakes easily with a fork and reaches an internal temperature of 145°F (63°C).

6. Serve the baked fish immediately, garnished with additional lemon wedges or fresh parsley if desired.

Tips:
- Adjust the baking time based on the thickness of your fish fillets. Thicker pieces may need an extra 2-3 minutes.

- For a crispy topping, sprinkle the fish with breadcrumbs or Parmesan cheese before baking.

- Try different herb and spice combinations, such as garlic, dill, or cajun seasoning.

- Bake the fish on a bed of sliced lemon, onion, or other vegetables for added flavor.

- Serve the baked fish with roasted potatoes, rice, or a fresh salad for a complete meal.

10. Cream of Rice Cereal

Ingredients:
- 1/2 cup (100g) cream of rice cereal
- 2 cups (480ml) milk or non-dairy milk
- 1/4 tsp salt
- 1-2 tbsp sugar, honey, or maple syrup (optional)

Instructions:

1. In a medium saucepan, whisk together the cream of rice cereal and milk.

2. Bring the mixture to a gentle simmer over medium heat, stirring frequently, until it begins to thicken, about 5-7 minutes.

3. Reduce the heat to low and continue cooking, stirring constantly, for an additional 5-10 minutes, until the cereal has a smooth, creamy consistency.

4. Remove the pan from the heat and stir in the salt. Taste and add sugar, honey, or maple syrup if desired, to sweeten the cereal to your liking.

5. Serve the cream of rice cereal warm, with any desired toppings such as fresh fruit, nuts, cinnamon, or a drizzle of additional milk.

Tips:
- For a thicker, creamier texture, use a 1:3 ratio of cream of rice to milk.

- Substitute non-dairy milk, such as almond, oat, or coconut milk, for a dairy-free version.

- Cook the cereal for a longer time to achieve a smoother, more porridge-like consistency.

- Stir in a spoonful of nut butter or cocoa powder for extra flavor.

- Top with fresh berries, sliced bananas, or a sprinkle of cinnamon or nutmeg.

- Refrigerate any leftover cereal and reheat it with a splash of milk when ready to serve.

11. Cottage Cheese

Cottage cheese is a versatile dairy product that can be enjoyed in a variety of ways. Here are some ideas for serving cottage cheese:

Plain:
- Serve cottage cheese on its own, either chilled or at room temperature. You can add a sprinkle of salt and pepper or a drizzle of honey for extra flavor.

With Fruit:
- Top cottage cheese with fresh or canned fruit, such as berries, peaches, pineapple, or melon.
- Try mixing in diced apples, grapes, or mandarin oranges.
- Sprinkle with a bit of cinnamon or a drizzle of maple syrup.

With Vegetables:
- Pair cottage cheese with sliced cucumbers, tomatoes, bell peppers, or radishes.
- Mix in diced avocado, shredded carrots, or chopped chives.

As a Dip:
- Use cottage cheese as a base for a savory dip, mixed with herbs, spices, or chopped vegetables.
- Serve with crackers, pita chips, or fresh veggies for dipping.

In Baked Goods:
- Fold cottage cheese into pancake or waffle batter for extra protein and moisture.
- Use it as a filling for crepes, blintzes, or stuffed French toast.
- Mix it into muffin or quick bread batters.

In Salads and Bowls:
- Add cottage cheese to green salads, grain bowls, or breakfast bowls for a protein boost.
- Mix it with quinoa, farro, or wild rice and top with roasted vegetables.

No matter how you choose to serve it, cottage cheese is a nutritious and versatile ingredient that can be enjoyed in both sweet and savory dishes.

12. Soft Tofu

Ingredients:
- 14 oz package soft or silken tofu
- 2 tbsp soy sauce or tamari
- 1 tbsp rice vinegar
- 1 tsp sesame oil
- 1 tsp grated ginger
- 2 green onions, sliced
- 1 tbsp toasted sesame seeds
- 2 tsp chili oil or chili crunch (optional)

Instructions:
1. Drain the tofu from the packaging and gently pat it dry with paper towels. Try not to break up the tofu block too much.

2. In a small bowl, whisk together the soy sauce, rice vinegar, sesame oil, and grated ginger.

3. Transfer the tofu to a shallow dish or plate. Pour the soy sauce mixture evenly over the top of the tofu, allowing it to soak in.

4. Sprinkle the sliced green onions and toasted sesame seeds over the top of the tofu.

5. If desired, drizzle some chili oil or chili crunch over the tofu for added heat and flavor.

6. Let the tofu marinate for 10-15 minutes to allow the flavors to soak in before serving.

7. Serve the soft tofu either chilled or at room temperature, along with rice, vegetables, or drizzled with additional soy sauce if desired.

Notes:
- Be very gentle when handling soft/silken tofu, as it can easily break apart.

- For added texture, you can dust the tofu lightly with cornstarch before marinating.

- Garnish with sliced cucumbers, radishes, or fresh herbs like cilantro or mint.

- Adjust soy sauce and vinegar amounts to taste preference.

- Try baking the marinated tofu for 15-20 minutes at 375°F for a warm preparation.

This soft tofu preparation allows the delicate texture to shine while adding wonderful savory, tangy, and umami flavors. It's a versatile dish that can be served warm or chilled.

13. Steamed Carrots

Ingredients:
- 1 lb carrots, peeled and cut into 1-inch pieces (or baby carrots)
- 1 tbsp butter or olive oil (optional)
- Salt and pepper to taste
- Chopped fresh parsley for garnish (optional)

Instructions:

1. Prepare the carrots by peeling them and cutting into 1-inch thick pieces or slices. If using baby carrots, you can leave them whole.

2. Fill a pot with 1-2 inches of water and insert a steamer basket. Bring the water to a boil over high heat.

3. Once the water is boiling, add the carrot pieces to the steamer basket in an even layer. Cover with a lid.

4. Steam the carrots for 8-12 minutes, depending on how crisp or tender you prefer them. Start checking at 8 minutes.

5. Once the carrots are fork-tender, remove the steamer basket from the pot using oven mitts.

6. Transfer the steamed carrots to a serving bowl. Toss with butter or olive oil if desired.

7. Season with salt and pepper to taste.

8. Optionally, garnish with chopped fresh parsley.

9. Serve the steamed carrots warm.

Notes:
- Add herbs like dill, thyme or garlic for extra flavor when steaming.
- For glazed carrots, toss with a glaze of maple syrup, brown sugar, honey, etc. after steaming.
- You can steam other veggies like broccoli, cauliflower, green beans etc using this method.
- Steaming helps retain more nutrients compared to boiling.

Steamed carrots make a simple, healthy and flavorful side dish. The bright orange color and tender-crisp texture are delightful!

14. Baked Chicken Breast

Ingredients:
- 4 boneless, skinless chicken breasts
- 2 tbsp olive oil or melted butter
- 1 tsp dried thyme
- 1 tsp dried rosemary
- 1 tsp paprika
- 1/2 tsp garlic powder
- Salt and pepper to taste

Instructions:
1. Preheat your oven to 400°F (200°C). Line a baking sheet with foil or parchment paper.

2. Pat the chicken breasts dry with paper towels and place them on the prepared baking sheet.

3. In a small bowl, combine the olive oil/melted butter, thyme, rosemary, paprika, garlic powder, salt and pepper.

4. Use a basting brush or spoon to evenly coat the chicken breasts with the seasoned oil/butter mixture on both sides.

5. Bake for 20-25 minutes, depending on the thickness, until the chicken is cooked through (165°F internal temperature).

6. For extra browning and crispness, you can optionally broil for 2-3 minutes at the end of cooking.

7. Allow the baked chicken breasts to rest for 5 minutes before serving.

8. Serve hot with desired sides like roasted veggies, rice, salad, etc. You can also slice or shred the chicken for other uses.

Notes:
- Feel free to adjust seasoning amounts to taste.
- Try adding lemon juice or zest, Italian seasoning or other dried herbs to the oil mixture.
- For an ultra juicy result, brine the chicken for 30 minutes to 1 hour before baking.
- Pound thicker breasts to ensure even cooking.
- Baste with pan juices occasionally while baking for more moisture.

Baked chicken breast is a versatile, lean protein that is easy to prepare. This simple spice mixture gives it delicious flavor!

15. Banana Smoothie

Ingredients:
- 2 ripe bananas
- 1 cup milk of your choice (dairy, almond, oat, etc.)
- 1/2 cup plain yogurt or Greek yogurt
- 2 tbsp honey or maple syrup (optional, for sweetness)
- 1 tsp vanilla extract
- 1 cup ice cubes

Instructions:

1. Peel the bananas and add them to a blender.

2. Pour in the milk and yogurt.

3. Add the honey/maple syrup if you want it sweeter. Also add the vanilla extract.

4. Add the ice cubes to the blender.

5. Blend on high speed for 1-2 minutes until completely smooth and frothy.

6. If it's too thick, add a splash more milk. If too thin, add more ice.

7. Once blended to your desired consistency, pour into glasses.

8. Optional toppings: sprinkle with cinnamon, nutmeg, granola, nut butter, etc.

9. Serve the banana smoothie immediately with a spoon or straw.

Notes:
- Use frozen banana chunks for an extra thick, frosty smoothie.
- For protein, add a scoop of protein powder or nut butter.
- Substitute Greek yogurt for a thicker, higher protein smoothie.
- Add greens like spinach or kale for extra nutrients.
- Use any milk you prefer - dairy, nut-milk, oat, etc.
- Top with coconut, chocolate chips or fresh fruit like berries.

This banana smoothie is cool, creamy and so satisfying! It's a great way to use up ripe bananas while getting protein, potassium and other nutrients. Perfect for breakfast or a snack.

16. Rice Pudding

Ingredients:
- 1/2 cup uncooked white rice (short or long grain)
- 2 cups milk (dairy or plant-based)
- 1/4 cup white sugar
- 1/4 tsp salt
- 1 egg, beaten
- 2 tbsp butter
- 1/2 tsp vanilla extract
- Ground cinnamon or nutmeg for dusting

Instructions:
1. In a saucepan, combine the uncooked rice, milk, sugar and salt. Bring to a simmer over medium heat, stirring frequently.

2. Once simmering, reduce heat to low and cook uncovered for 30-40 minutes, stirring occasionally, until the rice is very soft and most of the milk is absorbed.

3. In a small bowl, beat the egg. Temper it by stirring in a few spoonfuls of the hot rice mixture to prevent curdling.

4. Remove the saucepan from heat and stir in the tempered egg, butter and vanilla extract until fully incorporated.

5. Return saucepan to low heat and cook for 2-3 more minutes, stirring constantly, until thickened to your desired consistency.

6. Remove from heat and let cool slightly. The pudding will continue to thicken as it cools.

7. Portion into bowls or ramekins and dust the tops with ground cinnamon or nutmeg.

8. Serve the rice pudding warm or refrigerate until chilled through before serving.

Notes:
- For richer pudding, use half and half instead of milk.
- Add raisins, dried fruit, coconut or nuts if desired.
- Use brown sugar, honey or maple syrup in place of white sugar.
- Add vanilla bean or almond extract for extra flavor.
- Can use leftover cooked rice instead of uncooked.

This comforting, creamy rice pudding makes a wonderful dessert or snack. It's simple to prepare but so delicious!

17. Applesauce

Ingredients:
- 6-8 apples (a mix of sweet and tart varieties works well like Gala, Fuji, Granny Smith)
- 1/4 cup water or apple cider
- 1-2 tbsp white sugar or brown sugar (optional)
- 1 tsp ground cinnamon (optional)
- 1/4 tsp ground nutmeg (optional)

Instructions:

1. Peel, core, and slice the apples into rough 1-inch chunks.

2. In a saucepan, combine the apples and water/cider. Bring to a simmer over medium heat.

3. Cover and cook for 15-20 minutes, stirring occasionally, until apples are very soft and broken down.

4. Remove from heat and mash the apples to your desired consistency using a potato masher or immersion blender.

5. Stir in the sugar and spices if using. Adjust to taste.

6. Allow to cool slightly before serving warm or refrigerate until ready to eat.

Notes:
- For chunky applesauce, mash some but leave some pieces.

- For smoother sauce, blend more thoroughly or pass through a food mill.

- Add lemon juice to taste to brighten the flavor.

- Top with extra cinnamon or nutmeg if desired.

Homemade applesauce keeps refrigerated for 5-7 days. Enjoy as a snack, dessert topping or side dish!

18. Strained Fruit Juice

Ingredients:
- 2 lbs (1 kg) fresh fruit of your choice (e.g. strawberries, oranges, pineapple)
- 1/2 cup (120 ml) water or juice (optional)
- Honey or sugar to taste (optional)

Equipment Needed:
- Blender or food processor
- Fine mesh strainer or cheesecloth
- Bowl

Instructions:
1. Wash and prepare the fruit by removing any stems, cores, or rinds. Chop into chunks if needed.

2. In a blender or food processor, blend the fresh fruit with the water or juice (if using) until completely pureed and liquified.

3. Line a strainer or bowl with a few layers of cheesecloth. Pour the fruit puree into the lined strainer.

4. Using a spoon or ladle, gently press and stir the puree to help extract as much juice as possible through the strainer, leaving behind the pulp and solids.

5. Once strained, you can sweeten the juice with honey or sugar if desired. Start with 1-2 tablespoons and adjust to taste.

6. Transfer strained juice to a pitcher or jar. Refrigerate until ready to serve over ice or use in recipes.

Notes:
- Citrus fruits like oranges and grapefruits work great for juice. Berries, pineapple, mango also make tasty juices.

- For thicker juices from high-pulp fruits, you may need to strain it twice.

- Add water or juice to the pulp and re-strain to extract more juice if desired.

- Strained juices will keep refrigerated for 3-5 days.

You can drink the fresh juice as-is or use it in cocktails, smoothies, popsicles and more! Enjoy your homemade strained juice.

19. Turkey Deli Meat

Ingredients:
- 4 lbs boneless, skinless turkey breast
- 1/4 cup kosher salt
- 2 tbsp brown sugar
- 1 tsp black pepper
- 1 tsp garlic powder
- 1 tsp paprika
- 1/2 tsp curing salt
 (pink salt) - optional

Brine:
- 1 gallon water
- 1/2 cup kosher salt
- 1/2 cup brown sugar

Equipment:
- Meat grinder or sharp knife
- Smoker or oven
- Meat mallet or rolling pin

Instructions:

1. Make the brine by dissolving the salt and brown sugar in the water. Add the turkey and brine for 12-24 hours in the refrigerator.

2. Drain and pat the turkey dry. Discard the brine.

3. In a small bowl, mix together the salt, brown sugar, pepper, garlic, paprika and curing salt if using.

4. Lightly pound or roll the turkey breast to an even thickness of about 1/2 inch.

5. Rub the seasoning mixture all over the turkey breast on both sides.

6. For Smoking: Preheat smoker to 225°F with wood chips. Smoke for 2-3 hours until internal temp reaches 165°F.

7. For Oven: Place turkey on a foil-lined baking sheet. Bake at 250°F for 2-3 hours until 165°F internal temp.

8. Allow turkey to rest 15 minutes before slicing very thinly using a meat slicer, sharp knife or across the grain.

9. Layer the sliced turkey between parchment paper and press with a weight for 30-60 minutes to compress it deli-style.

10. Refrigerate deli turkey slices for up to 1 week or freeze for longer storage.

Serve the homemade turkey deli meat on sandwiches, wraps, or enjoy plain. Adjust the smoke time and seasonings to your taste preferences.

20. White Rice Congee

Ingredients:
- 1 cup long grain white rice
- 8 cups chicken or vegetable broth
- ¼ tsp salt (or to taste)
- White pepper to taste
- Toppings: green onions, fried shallots, pork floss, soy sauce, sesame oil, etc. (optional)

Instructions:

1. Rinse the rice until the water runs clear. Drain well.

2. In a large pot, combine the rinsed rice and broth. Bring to a boil over high heat.

3. Once boiling, reduce heat to low, cover and simmer for 1 hour, stirring occasionally to prevent sticking or scorching.

4. After 1 hour, the congee should have a thick, porridge-like consistency. If still too thin, cook uncovered for 10-15 minutes more until thickened.

5. Season the congee with salt and white pepper to taste.

6. Ladle the hot congee into bowls. Add desired toppings like green onions, fried shallots, pork floss, soy sauce or sesame oil.

Notes:

- For thicker texture, use up to 10 cups of broth and increase simmering time.

- For variation, cook the rice with chicken stock instead of broth.

- Add meat like shredded chicken or sliced century eggs to make it heartier.

- Leftover congee will continue to thicken as it cools. Add broth to thin it out when reheating.

Congee is a savory rice porridge that is a classic comfort food in many Asian cuisines. This plain white congee makes a great base to customize with your favorite savory toppings and mix-ins. Enjoy!

21. Low-Fiber Cereal

Ingredients:
- 1 cup white rice flour
- 1/2 cup tapioca flour
- 1/2 cup potato starch
- 1 tsp salt
- 1 tsp sugar (optional)
- 2 tbsp butter or oil
- 1/2 cup milk or milk alternative
- 1 egg, beaten

For Coating:
- 1 tbsp butter or oil
- 1/4 cup white sugar (optional)
- 1 tsp cinnamon (optional)

Instructions:

1. In a large bowl, whisk together the white rice flour, tapioca flour, potato starch, salt and sugar if using.

2. Make a well in the center and pour in the butter/oil and milk. Mix together until a soft dough forms.

3. Turn dough onto a lightly floured surface and knead for 2-3 minutes until smooth and combined.

4. Roll or pat the dough into a rectangle about 1/4 inch thick.

5. Using a pizza cutter or knife, cut the dough into small square pieces.

6. In a shallow bowl, beat the egg with a splash of water or milk. In another bowl, mix the sugar and cinnamon if using.

7. Dip each cereal piece first into the egg wash, then into the cinnamon-sugar coating if desired.

8. Place coated pieces spaced apart on a parchment lined baking sheet.

9. Bake at 350°F for 10-12 minutes until lightly golden brown.

10. Allow to cool completely before storing in an airtight container for up to 2 weeks.

These crispy low-fiber cereal pieces are perfect for those on a low residue diet. Serve with milk, dairy-free milk or yogurt. The coating is optional if you want to reduce the sugar content further.

22. Creamy Peanut Butter

Ingredients:
- 2 cups roasted unsalted peanuts
- 1-2 tsp peanut oil or vegetable oil
- 1/2 tsp salt (optional)
- 1-2 tsp honey or maple syrup (optional)

Equipment Needed: Food processor or high-powered blender

Instructions:

1. Pour the roasted peanuts into the bowl of a food processor or blender.

2. Process the peanuts for 1 minute, stopping to scrape down the sides as needed. The peanuts should look dry and crumbly at this point.

3. Continue processing for another 2-3 minutes, stopping to scrape down the sides frequently. The peanut butter will go through stages from dry crumbs, to a dry ball, and then it will gradually start releasing its oils and turning creamy.

4. Once the peanut butter looks smooth and creamy, with just a few tiny pieces of peanuts remaining, you can stop processing if you like a slightly crunchy texture. For super creamy peanut butter, process 1-2 minutes more.

5. With the machine running, drizzle in 1-2 tsp of peanut or vegetable oil through the feed tube to help it along if needed. The oil helps reach that ultra creamy texture.

6. Finally, add salt to taste (about 1/2 tsp) and/or honey/maple syrup (1-2 tsp) if you want a touch of sweetness.

7. Process briefly to incorporate the add-ins. Then transfer to an airtight container.

That's it! Store the homemade creamy peanut butter at room temperature for up to 2 months. Stir before using if oil separates. Enjoy on bread, in baking, or straight from the jar!

23. Plain Bagels

Ingredients:
- 1 cup (240ml) warm water
- 1 tbsp (12g) sugar
- 1 tsp salt

For Boiling:
- 4 quarts (4 liters) water
- 1 tbsp sugar or malt powder

- 1 tbsp (8g) active dry yeast
- 3 1/4 cups (390g) bread flour or high protein flour
- 1 egg white, beaten with 1 tbsp water for egg wash
- Toppings like sesame seeds, poppy seeds, etc (optional)

Instructions:

1. In a large bowl, combine the warm water, sugar, salt and yeast. Let sit for 5 minutes until frothy.

2. Add in 3 cups of the flour and stir with a wooden spoon until a shaggy dough forms.

3. Turn out onto a lightly floured surface and knead for 8-10 minutes, working in remaining 1/4 cup flour as needed until dough is smooth and elastic.

4. Place dough in a lightly greased bowl, cover and let rise for 1 hour or until doubled in size.

5. Punch down the dough to release air bubbles. Divide into 8 equal pieces.

6. Roll each piece into a smooth ball. Use your thumb to punch a hole in the center and stretch into a bagel shape, rotating and stretching to form an even ring.

7. In a large pot, bring the 4 quarts of water and 1 tbsp sugar/malt powder to a boil.

8. Carefully add 2-3 bagels at a time and boil for 1 minute per side.

9. Remove boiled bagels with a slotted spoon and place on a parchment-lined baking sheet.

10. Brush the bagel tops with the egg wash and sprinkle with desired toppings if using.

11. Bake at 425°F for 20-25 minutes until deeply golden brown.

12. Allow to cool slightly before serving warm or at room temperature.

For an extra chewy bagel, let the boiled and topped bagels rest for 20 minutes before baking. Enjoy these fresh homemade plain bagels for breakfast or anytime!

24. Vanilla Pudding

Ingredients:
- 1/2 cup (100g) white granulated sugar
- 1/4 cup (30g) cornstarch
- 1/4 tsp salt
- 2 cups (475ml) whole milk
- 2 large eggs
- 2 tbsp (28g) unsalted butter
- 2 tsp vanilla extract

Instructions:
1. In a medium saucepan, whisk together the sugar, cornstarch, and salt. Gradually whisk in the milk until fully combined.

2. Crack the eggs into a small bowl and beat lightly. Scoop out about 1/4 cup of the milk mixture and gradually whisk it into the beaten eggs to temper them.

3. Pour the egg mixture back into the saucepan with the remaining milk mixture and whisk to combine fully.

4. Cook over medium heat, whisking frequently, until the mixture begins to bubble and thicken, about 5-8 minutes.

5. Once it reaches a pudding-like thickness, remove from heat and whisk in the butter and vanilla extract until fully incorporated.

6. Pour the pudding into a bowl or individual ramekins. Cover with plastic wrap pressed directly onto the surface to prevent a skin from forming.

7. Refrigerate for at least 2 hours before serving to allow it to set up fully.

8. When ready to serve, you can top with whipped cream, crushed cookies, chocolate shavings or enjoy plain.

Notes:
- For extra richness, substitute half-and-half or cream for some of the milk.
- Add a pinch of cinnamon or nutmeg for extra flavor if desired.
- Pudding will continue to thicken as it cools completely in the fridge.

This classic homemade vanilla pudding makes a simple yet delicious dessert or snack. Enjoy chilled or at room temperature.

25. White Bread Rolls

Ingredients:
- 1 cup (240ml) warm milk
- 1 tbsp (12g) granulated sugar
- 1 packet (7g) active dry yeast
- 3 cups (375g) all-purpose flour
- 1 tsp salt
- 2 tbsp (28g) unsalted butter, softened
- 1 egg, lightly beaten with 1 tbsp water (for egg wash)

Instructions:

1. In a small bowl, combine the warm milk, sugar and yeast. Let sit for 5-10 minutes until frothy.

2. In a large bowl, whisk together the flour and salt. Create a well in the middle.

3. Pour in the yeast mixture and softened butter. Use a wooden spoon to stir everything together into a shaggy dough.

4. Turn dough onto a lightly floured surface and knead for 5-7 minutes, until smooth and elastic. Form into a ball.

5. Place dough in a lightly greased bowl, cover with plastic wrap or towel, and let rise for 1 hour or until doubled in size.

6. Punch down the dough to release air bubbles. On a lightly floured surface, divide dough into 12 equal pieces.

7. Shape each piece into a smooth ball by pulling the edges under and pinching to seal on the bottom. Place on a parchment-lined baking sheet, spacing them about 2 inches apart.

8. Cover and let rise for 30 minutes. Meanwhile, preheat oven to 375°F. Brush the tops of the rolls with the egg wash mixture.

9. Bake for 15-18 minutes until golden brown on top. Remove from oven and brush tops with melted butter if desired. Allow rolls to cool slightly before serving warm.

These soft, fluffy white bread rolls make a great accompaniment to meals or can be used for sliders or sandwiches. Enjoy the homemade rolls fresh out of the oven!

26. Boiled Eggs

Ingredients:
- Eggs (as many as needed)
- Water for boiling
- Salt (optional)

Equipment:
- Saucepan with lid
- Slotted spoon
- Bowl of ice water (for easy peeling)

Instructions:
1. Place the eggs in a single layer in a saucepan and cover with cold water by 1 inch.

2. Add a pinch of salt to the water if desired (it helps prevent cracking).

3. Bring the water to a rapid boil over high heat.

4. Once boiling, remove the pan from heat, cover with a lid and let stand:
    - Soft boiled: 6-7 minutes
    - Hard boiled: 12 minutes

5. Prepare an ice water bath by filling a bowl with cold water and ice cubes.

6. When time is up, use a slotted spoon to transfer the eggs from the hot water to the ice bath to stop the cooking process.

7. Let the eggs sit in the ice bath for 5 minutes before peeling.

8. To peel, gently tap the wider end of the egg on a hard surface to crack the shell all over. Start peeling from the air pocket at the wider end.

9. Rinse peeled eggs under cold water to wash away any shell fragments.

For Easy Peeling:
- Use older eggs (7-10 days old) rather than super fresh eggs
- Add a teaspoon of baking soda to the boiling water

That's it! You can enjoy the boiled eggs right away while warm, or refrigerate them for snacks, salads or deviled eggs later. Adjust the boiling time up or down for your desired yolk consistency.

27. Fish Fillet Sandwich

Ingredients:
- 1 tsp garlic powder
- Salt and pepper to taste
- Vegetable oil for frying
- 4 burger buns
- Tartar sauce
- Lettuce, tomato, onion (optional toppings)
- 4 white fish fillets (cod, tilapia, etc), about 6 oz each
- 1 cup all-purpose flour
- 2 eggs, beaten
- 1 1/2 cups panko breadcrumbs
- 1 tsp paprika

Instructions:

1. Rinse the fish fillets and pat them dry with paper towels. Season both sides with salt and pepper.

2. Set up three shallow dishes - one with flour, one with beaten eggs, and one with panko breadcrumbs mixed with paprika and garlic powder.

3. Dredge each fillet first in the flour, dip in the egg, and then coat completely with the seasoned panko crumbs, pressing gently to adhere.

4. Pour vegetable oil about 1/2 inch deep in a skillet and heat over medium-high heat to 350°F.

5. Fry the breaded fillets 2-3 at a time for 2-3 minutes per side until golden brown and crispy. Drain on a wire rack.

6. Toast or grill the burger buns until lightly browned if desired.

7. Spread tartar sauce on both bun halves. Add lettuce, tomato, onion if using.

8. Place a fried fish fillet on each bottom bun and top with the other bun half.

9. Serve the fish sandwiches immediately while the fish is hot and crispy.

Some tasty extras:
- Malt vinegar or lemon wedges for squeezing over the fish
- Pickles or coleslaw on the sandwich
- Swiss, cheddar or pepper jack cheese melted on the fish

Crispy fried fish fillets make such a satisfying sandwich! Adjust cooking time as needed based on thickness of the fillets.

28. Grilled Chicken Breast

Ingredients:
- 4 boneless, skinless chicken breasts
- 2 tbsp olive oil
- 1 tsp kosher salt
- 1/2 tsp black pepper
- 1/2 tsp garlic powder
- 1/2 tsp paprika
- 1/4 tsp cayenne pepper (optional)

For Basting (optional):
- 2 tbsp butter, melted
- 1 tbsp fresh herbs (thyme, rosemary, etc)

Instructions:
1. Take the chicken breasts out of the packaging and pat them dry with paper towels. Use a meat mallet to gently pound the thicker parts of the breast to an even thickness of about 3/4 inch. This allows for even cooking.

2. In a small bowl, mix together the olive oil, salt, pepper, garlic powder, paprika, and cayenne if using.

3. Brush or rub the seasoning mixture over all sides of the chicken breasts.

4. Prepare grill for direct cooking over medium-high heat (375-450°F).

5. Place chicken breasts on the hot grill grates. Cover and cook for 5-7 minutes per side, flipping only once, until the internal temperature reaches 160°F.

6. If basting, use a brush to baste the chicken with the melted herb butter during the final few minutes of cooking.

7. Remove chicken from the grill once it reaches an internal temperature of 165°F. Allow the chicken to rest for 5 minutes before slicing or serving.

Some tips:
- Cook over direct, high heat to get great grill marks
- Use a meat thermometer to avoid overcooking
- Brine the chicken for extra juiciness if desired
- Let rest to allow juices to reincorporate

29. Cheese Omelette

Ingredients:
- 3 large eggs
- 1 tbsp water or milk
- 1/4 tsp salt
- 1/8 tsp black pepper
- 1 tbsp butter
- 1/2 cup shredded cheddar or your favorite cheese
- Optional fillings: diced ham, bacon, veggies, herbs, etc.

Instructions:

1. Crack the eggs into a small bowl and beat them lightly with a fork. Add the water/milk, salt and pepper and beat to incorporate.

2. Melt the butter in an 8-inch nonstick skillet over medium heat, swirling to coat the pan.

3. Pour in the beaten eggs and let them sit for 10-15 seconds to set the bottom lightly.

4. Using a spatula, gently push the eggs from the side of the pan into the center, tilting the pan to allow the uncooked egg to flow to the edge.

5. When the bottom is set but the top is still moist, sprinkle on the shredded cheese and any other fillings you want over half of the omelette.

6. Let cook for 30 seconds more until the cheese is slightly melted.

7. Fold the plain half over the filled half using the spatula. Slide the folded omelette onto a plate.

8. Serve the cheese omelette immediately while hot.

Some tasty filling ideas:
- Diced ham, bacon, sausage
- Sauteed mushrooms, spinach, tomatoes, onions
- Salsa, avocado
- Fresh herbs like chives, parsley, dill

The perfect cheese omelette has melt-y cheese layered inside light, fluffy eggs. Feel free to get creative with fillings or just enjoy it plain. Breakfast is served!

30. Creamy Polenta

Ingredients:
- 4 cups water or broth (chicken, veggie)
- 1 tsp salt
- 1 cup polenta/cornmeal
- 3 tbsp butter
- 1/2 cup grated parmesan cheese
- 1/4 cup heavy cream or milk
- Black pepper to taste

Instructions:

1. In a medium saucepan, bring the water or broth to a boil over high heat. Add the salt.

2. Once boiling, slowly pour in the polenta while whisking constantly to prevent lumps.

3. Reduce heat to low and continue simmering, stirring frequently with a wooden spoon or whisk every few minutes. Cook for 20-25 minutes until thickened to a porridge-like consistency.

4. Remove the polenta from heat and stir in the butter until melted and incorporated.

5. Next, stir in the grated parmesan and heavy cream until fully combined. The mixture should be very creamy.

6. Taste and season with black pepper and additional salt if needed.

7. For a thinner polenta, stir in a few more splashes of cream or broth until desired consistency is reached.

8. Serve the creamy polenta immediately while hot, garnished with extra parmesan if desired.

Some ways to serve polenta:
- As a side with roasted meats, stews, sauces
- Pour into a baking dish, let set, then slice and fry or grill
- Stir in sauteed mushrooms, greens, sun-dried tomatoes
- Top with a poached egg

This classic Italian porridge made from cornmeal is so versatile! The parmesan and cream make it luxuriously smooth and flavorful.

31. Custard

Ingredients:
- 4 large egg yolks
- 1/3 cup (65g) granulated sugar
- 1/4 tsp salt
- 2 cups (475ml) whole milk
- 1 tsp vanilla extract
- Freshly grated nutmeg (optional)

Instructions:
1. In a medium bowl, whisk together the egg yolks, sugar, and salt until light and fluffy.

2. In a saucepan, heat the milk over medium just until steaming and bubbles start to form around the edges. Do not boil.

3. Temper the egg yolks by slowly pouring 1/2 cup of the hot milk into the yolk mixture while whisking constantly.

4. Then slowly whisk the tempered yolk mixture back into the saucepan with the remaining hot milk.

5. Cook over medium-low heat, stirring constantly with a wooden spoon or heat-proof spatula, until thickened enough to coat the back of the spoon, about 5-7 minutes. Do not boil.

6. Remove from heat and stir in the vanilla extract.

7. Strain the custard through a fine mesh sieve into a bowl or ramekins to remove any possible scrambled egg pieces.

8. Press plastic wrap directly on the surface to prevent a skin from forming. Refrigerate for at least 2 hours until chilled and set. When ready to serve, grate fresh nutmeg over the top if desired.

Tips:
- For richer custard, use more egg yolks or some heavy cream in place of some milk
- Eat custard within 3-4 days refrigerated
- Add flavorings like vanilla bean, cinnamon, coffee, etc.
- Serve with fresh berries, caramel sauce, whipped cream

This classic custard makes a simple but luxurious dessert, pie filling, or base for other custard dishes. Rich, creamy, and perfect when chilled.

32. Smooth Peanut Butter Sandwich

Ingredients:
- 2 slices of bread (any type you prefer)
- 2-3 tablespoons creamy peanut butter
- Optional extras: sliced bananas, honey, jelly/jam

Instructions:

1. Take the two slices of bread and lay them flat on a cutting board or plate.

2. Use a butter knife to spread an even layer of creamy peanut butter over one slice of bread. Use as much or as little peanut butter as you like.

3. If adding any extras like sliced bananas or honey, layer them on top of the peanut butter on that slice.

4. Place the other plain slice of bread on top to form a sandwich.

5. Press down gently to allow the peanut butter to adhere to both slices.

6. Cut the sandwich in half diagonally or leave it whole.

7. Enjoy your classic, creamy peanut butter sandwich!

You can use crunchy peanut butter instead of smooth if you prefer that texture. Peanut butter and jelly/jam is another popular variety where you spread jelly on one slice before assembling.

33. Plain Yogurt

Ingredients:
- 4 cups (1 liter) whole milk
- 1/4 cup (60ml) plain yogurt with live active cultures

Equipment:
- Saucepan
- Candy/food thermometer
- Yogurt maker or thermal container to incubate

Instructions:

1. Heat the milk: Pour the milk into a saucepan and heat over medium, stirring frequently, until it reaches 180°F (82°C). This pasteurizes the milk.

2. Cool the milk: Allow the milk to cool to 110-115°F (43-46°C). You can speed this up by placing the pan in an ice water bath and stirring frequently.

3. Add yogurt starter: Transfer some of the warm milk into a bowl and whisk in the 1/4 cup plain yogurt until fully incorporated. This is the yogurt starter.

4. Combine: Pour the yogurt starter mixture back into the remaining warm milk and whisk to fully combine.

5. Incubate: Pour the milk-yogurt mixture into a yogurt maker or thermal insulated container. Incubate at 110°F (43°C) for 6-12 hours, until it has set into yogurt.

6. Refrigerate: Once set, refrigerate the yogurt. It will continue to thicken as it chills.

You can adjust thickness by straining some of the whey off for a thicker Greek-style yogurt. Add a bit of milk to thin it out if desired.

Enjoy your fresh, tangy plain yogurt! It's delicious on its own, with fruit, granola or in recipes. The active cultures make it a probiotic food.

34. Macaroni and Cheese

Ingredients:
- 8 oz (225g) elbow macaroni or other short pasta
- 4 tbsp (55g) butter
- 1/4 cup (30g) all-purpose flour
- 2 cups (480ml) milk
- 1/2 tsp salt
- 1/4 tsp black pepper
- 1/4 tsp paprika
- 2 cups (225g) shredded cheddar cheese
- 1/2 cup (55g) shredded parmesan cheese

Instructions:

1. Cook the pasta: Bring a large pot of salted water to a boil. Add the macaroni and cook according to package instructions until al dente. Drain and set aside.

2. Make the cheese sauce: In a saucepan, melt the butter over medium heat. Whisk in the flour and cook for 1 minute. Gradually whisk in the milk. Cook until thickened, about 5 minutes.

3. Season the sauce: Remove from heat and stir in the salt, pepper, paprika, 1 1/2 cups cheddar cheese and 1/4 cup parmesan. Stir until the cheese melts and the sauce is smooth.

4. Combine pasta and sauce: Add the cooked macaroni to the cheese sauce and stir to coat the pasta evenly.

5. Transfer to baking dish: Transfer the macaroni and cheese to a lightly greased 2-quart baking dish. Top with remaining 1/2 cup cheddar and 1/4 cup parmesan.

6. Bake: Bake at 350°F (175°C) for 20-25 minutes until hot and the top is golden brown.

Let the macaroni and cheese rest for 5 minutes before serving. For an extra crispy top, you can switch the oven to broil for 2-3 minutes at the end.

Creamy, cheesy and delicious! This homemade version is sure to be a hit. You can add extras like breadcrumbs, bacon or roasted veggies if desired.

35. Rice Noodles Soup

Ingredients:
- 8 oz (225g) thin rice noodles (or rice stick noodles)
- 6 cups (1.4 liters) chicken or vegetable broth
- 2 cups (480ml) water
- 2 cloves garlic, minced
- 1 inch (2.5cm) ginger, grated or minced
- 2 tbsp soy sauce
- 1 tbsp rice vinegar
- 1 tsp sesame oil
- Sliced green onions or chives
- Other toppings: shredded chicken, mushrooms, bean sprouts, chili oil etc.

Instructions:

1. Soak the rice noodles in hot water for 10-15 minutes until pliable but still undercooked. Drain and set aside.

2. In a large pot, combine the broth, water, garlic, ginger, soy sauce, rice vinegar and sesame oil. Bring to a boil.

3. Add the soaked rice noodles and any proteins or veggies you want in the soup (like shredded chicken and mushrooms).

4. Simmer for 3-5 minutes until the noodles are cooked through and ingredients are heated.

5. Remove from heat and add in any fresh toppings like green onions and bean sprouts.

6. Ladle the hot soup into bowls and serve immediately with chili oil or other toppings on the side if desired.

The great thing about this soup is you can customize it by adding your favorite proteins like shrimp or beef. Or keep it vegetarian with just veggies.

The thin rice noodles soak up all the delicious savory broth flavors. It's light yet satisfying and makes a perfect lunch or dinner soup.

36. Chicken Salad with Mayo

Ingredients:
- 2 cups cooked chicken, shredded or chopped
- 1/2 cup mayonnaise
- 1 stalk celery, diced
- 2 green onions, sliced
- 2 tbsp lemon juice
- 1 tsp Dijon mustard
- 1/4 tsp each salt and pepper
- Optional add-ins: sliced grapes, dried cranberries, chopped nuts

Instructions:

1. In a large bowl, combine the cooked chicken, mayonnaise, celery, green onions, lemon juice, mustard, salt and pepper.

2. Mix everything together until well combined and the chicken is evenly coated in the mayonnaise dressing.

3. Taste and adjust seasonings as needed, adding more mayo for extra creaminess if desired.

4. If using any extra add-ins like grapes, dried cranberries or nuts, gently fold them in now.

5. Cover and refrigerate for at least 30 minutes to allow flavors to meld.

6. Serve the chicken salad on a bed of lettuce, in a sandwich, wrap or with crackers. Garnish with extra green onion if desired.

This chicken salad is cool, creamy and so flavorful from the mayonnaise dressing. The celery adds great crunch while the lemon juice brightens it up. Feel free to add your favorite extras like dried fruit or nuts.

It's a great way to use up leftover cooked chicken and makes a perfect lunch, snack or light dinner. Enjoy!

37. Roasted Chicken Thighs

Ingredients:
- 8 bone-in, skin-on chicken thighs
- 2 tbsp olive oil
- 1 tsp salt
- 1/2 tsp black pepper
- 1 tsp paprika
- 1 tsp garlic powder
- 1 tsp dried thyme (or other herb like rosemary)

Instructions:

1. Pat the chicken thighs dry with paper towels and place them in a large bowl.

2. In a small bowl, combine the olive oil, salt, pepper, paprika, garlic powder and dried thyme.

3. Pour the olive oil mixture over the chicken thighs and use your hands to rub it all over, making sure the thighs are evenly coated in the seasoning.

4. Arrange the chicken thighs skin-side up on a rimmed baking sheet lined with foil or parchment paper.

5. Roast at 400°F (200°C) for 35-40 minutes, until the chicken is cooked through and the skin is crispy and golden brown.

6. Transfer the roasted thighs to a plate and let rest for 5 minutes before serving.

7. Optionally, you can make a quick pan sauce by deglazing the baking sheet with a splash of chicken broth or white wine while scraping up any browned bits. Pour the sauce over the chicken.

These roasted chicken thighs are incredibly juicy on the inside with crispy, flavorful skin. The simple seasoning blend gives them great savory flavor.

Serve the thighs alongside roasted veggies, mashed potatoes or a salad for a delicious meal. The leftovers also make great chicken salad or soup additions later in the week.

38. Soft Scrambled Tofu

Ingredients:
- 1 (14 oz) block extra-firm tofu, drained and crumbled
- 2 tbsp olive oil or vegan butter
- 1/4 cup unsweetened plant-based milk (like almond or soy milk)
- 1 tsp turmeric
- 1 tsp garlic powder
- 1 tsp onion powder
- 1/2 tsp salt
- 1/4 tsp black pepper
- 2 tbsp nutritional yeast (optional)
- Chopped scallions or chives for garnish

Instructions:

1. In a bowl, use your hands to crumble the drained tofu into a scrambled egg-like texture. Try to avoid overly mashing it.

2. Heat the oil/vegan butter in a non-stick skillet over medium heat.

3. Add the crumbled tofu and spices (turmeric, garlic powder, onion powder, salt, pepper). Gently stir to coat the tofu in the spices.

4. Pour in the plant-based milk and continue cooking for 2-3 minutes, gently folding the mixture with a spatula to incorporate the milk and prevent browning.

5. Once heated through, stir in the nutritional yeast if using for an eggy, savory flavor boost.

6. Remove from heat and optionally stir in some chopped scallions or chives.

7. Serve the soft scrambled tofu immediately, either plain or in a tortilla, on toast, etc.

The keys are using extra-firm tofu crumbled but not overly mashed, and cooking gently to create a soft, creamy scrambled texture. The turmeric gives it a golden yellow color like eggs.

This scrambled tofu makes a delicious, protein-packed vegan breakfast or brunch dish. Adjust spice levels to your taste preferences.

39. White Rice Risotto

Ingredients:
- 6 cups chicken or vegetable broth
- 3 tbsp olive oil
- 1 cup arborio rice
- 1/2 cup dry white wine (optional)
- 1 shallot, finely chopped
- 2 garlic cloves, minced
- 1/2 cup grated parmesan cheese
- 2 tbsp butter
- Salt and pepper to taste
- Chopped parsley for garnish

Instructions:
1. In a saucepan, warm the broth over low heat.

2. Heat the olive oil in a large skillet or pot over medium heat. Add the shallot and garlic and cook for 1 minute until fragrant.

3. Add the arborio rice and stir to coat with the oil. Cook for 2-3 minutes to lightly toast the rice.

4. Pour in the white wine (if using) and cook, stirring frequently, until absorbed.

5. Begin adding the warm broth 1/2 cup at a time, stirring frequently. Wait until the liquid is mostly absorbed before adding the next 1/2 cup.

6. Continue this process for 18-22 minutes, until the rice is cooked through but still has a slight bite. Add more broth as needed.

7. Remove from heat and stir in the parmesan and butter until melted and creamy.

8. Season with salt and pepper to taste.

9. Garnish with chopped parsley and serve immediately while warm.

The key to making risotto is slowly incorporating the warm broth while stirring frequently to release the rice's starches for a creamy texture.

You can add other ingredients like sauteed mushrooms, peas, crispy prosciutto or lemon zest. But this basic parmesan version lets the rice shine.

40. Soft Cheese

Ingredients:
- 6 cups chicken or vegetable broth
- 3 tbsp olive oil
- 1 cup arborio rice
- 1/2 cup dry white wine (optional)
- 1 shallot, finely chopped
- 2 garlic cloves, minced
- 1/2 cup grated parmesan cheese
- 2 tbsp butter
- Salt and pepper to taste
- Chopped parsley for garnish

Instructions:
1. In a saucepan, warm the broth over low heat.

2. Heat the olive oil in a large skillet or pot over medium heat. Add the shallot and garlic and cook for 1 minute until fragrant.

3. Add the arborio rice and stir to coat with the oil. Cook for 2-3 minutes to lightly toast the rice.

4. Pour in the white wine (if using) and cook, stirring frequently, until absorbed.

5. Begin adding the warm broth 1/2 cup at a time, stirring frequently. Wait until the liquid is mostly absorbed before adding the next 1/2 cup.

6. Continue this process for 18-22 minutes, until the rice is cooked through but still has a slight bite. Add more broth as needed.

7. Remove from heat and stir in the parmesan and butter until melted and creamy.

8. Season with salt and pepper to taste.

9. Garnish with chopped parsley and serve immediately while warm.

The key to making risotto is slowly incorporating the warm broth while stirring frequently to release the rice's starches for a creamy texture.

You can add other ingredients like sauteed mushrooms, peas, crispy prosciutto or lemon zest. But this basic parmesan version lets the rice shine.

41. Creamy Tomato Soup

Ingredients:
- 2 tbsp olive oil
- 1 onion, diced
- 3 garlic cloves, minced
- 2 (28oz) cans diced tomatoes
- 2 cups vegetable or chicken broth
- 1 cup heavy cream or half-and-half
- 1/4 cup fresh basil leaves, plus more for garnish
- 1 tsp dried oregano
- 1/2 tsp sugar
- Salt and pepper to taste

Instructions:
1. In a large pot or dutch oven, heat the olive oil over medium heat. Add the diced onion and cook for 5 minutes until softened.

2. Add the minced garlic and cook for 1 minute until fragrant.

3. Pour in the canned diced tomatoes with their juices, and the vegetable/chicken broth.

4. Add the basil leaves, dried oregano, sugar, and season with salt and pepper to taste.

5. Bring the soup to a simmer and let simmer for 15-20 minutes to allow flavors to meld.

6. Remove the basil leaves. Use an immersion blender to puree the soup until smooth, or puree in batches in a blender.

7. Once smooth, stir in the heavy cream or half-and-half until fully incorporated.

8. Taste and adjust seasoning if needed, adding more salt/pepper/sugar to your preferences.

9. Serve the creamy tomato soup garnished with extra basil leaves, croutons, parmesan, etc if desired.

This soup is so rich, velvety and full of tomatoey flavor. The cream adds such an indulgent creaminess. Perfect for dunking grilled cheese!

You can use fresh tomatoes instead of canned when in season. Adding a parmesan rind to the simmering soup is another way to add great depth of flavor.

42. Rice Cake with Cream Cheese

Ingredients:
- 4-6 plain rice cakes
- 4 oz (113g) cream cheese, softened
- 1 tbsp milk or water (optional)
- Salt and pepper to taste
- Toppings of choice: sliced cucumbers, tomatoes, smoked salmon, everything bagel seasoning, fresh herbs, etc.

Instructions:

1. If the cream cheese is very firm, let it soften at room temperature for 30 minutes to 1 hour until spreadable.

2. In a small bowl, mix together the softened cream cheese with 1 tbsp of milk or water until you reach a nice spreadable consistency. You may not need any liquid if your cream cheese was very soft already.

3. Season the cream cheese mixture with a pinch of salt and pepper, or any other desired seasonings like dill, garlic powder, etc.

4. Spread an even layer of the seasoned cream cheese mixture on top of each rice cake.

5. Top the cream cheese with any desired toppings like sliced cucumbers, tomatoes, smoked salmon, everything bagel seasoning, fresh herbs, etc.

6. Enjoy the rice cakes right away for the best texture and flavor.

These make a great snack or light breakfast/lunch. The rice cakes provide a crispy, neutral base to pile on the creamy, tangy cream cheese and fun toppings.

For added protein, you can mix the cream cheese with smashed avocado or hummus. The topping possibilities are endless! Just be sure to eat them soon after assembling for maximum freshness.

43. Steamed White Fish

Ingredients:
- 4 (6 oz) white fish fillets (cod, tilapia, halibut, etc)
- 2 tbsp olive oil or butter
- 2 cloves garlic, minced
- Juice of 1 lemon
- Salt and pepper to taste
- Chopped parsley for garnish

For Steaming:
- Steamer basket
- Pot with a tight-fitting lid

Instructions:
1. Pat the fish fillets dry with paper towels and season both sides with salt, pepper, and half the minced garlic.

2. In a small bowl, mix together the olive oil/melted butter, lemon juice, and remaining minced garlic.

3. Add 1-2 inches of water to the bottom of the pot and insert the steamer basket. Bring the water to a simmer over high heat.

4. Place the fish fillets in a single layer in the steamer basket, folding thin ends under to ensure even cooking.

5. Once simmering, pour half the lemon-garlic mixture over the fish.

6. Cover with a tight-fitting lid and steam for 8-12 minutes until the fish is opaque and flakes easily with a fork. Thicker fillets may need a couple more minutes.

7. Carefully remove the steamed fish and transfer to a platter. Drizzle the remaining lemon-garlic sauce over top.

8. Garnish with chopped parsley and lemon wedges if desired. Serve immediately.

Steaming is a gentle, healthy way to cook fish while keeping it moist and delicate in texture. The garlic, lemon, and herbs add lovely fresh flavors.

Feel free to swap the white fish for your favorite variety like salmon, sea bass, or snapper. Adjust steaming time as needed based on thickness.

44. Vanilla Milkshake

Ingredients:
- 2 cups vanilla ice cream
- 1 cup cold milk
- 1 tsp vanilla extract
- Whipped cream and cherry for garnish (optional)

Instructions:

1. Take the ice cream out of the freezer and allow it to sit at room temperature for 5-10 minutes to soften slightly.

2. In a blender, combine the slightly softened vanilla ice cream, cold milk, and vanilla extract.

3. Blend on high speed for 30 seconds - 1 minute until thick, creamy and combined. Scrape down sides as needed.

4. For an extra thick milkshake, use less milk or add a couple extra scoops of ice cream.

5. Pour the milkshake into a tall glass.

6. Top with whipped cream, a cherry, or any other fun toppings like sprinkles, chocolate syrup, etc. if desired.

7. Serve the milkshake immediately with a straw and a long spoon.

The keys are to use high quality ice cream and to leave it slightly soft before blending so it incorporates fully with the milk. The vanilla adds incredible flavor.

You can easily change up the flavor by using a different ice cream like chocolate, strawberry or coffee. Have fun experimenting with mix-ins too like peanut butter or malt powder.

This thick, creamy, icy cold milkshake is such a classic diner-style treat. Pure nostalgia in a glass!

45. Turkey and Cheese Sandwich

Ingredients:
- 2 slices bread (sourdough, whole wheat, etc.)
- 2-3 slices deli turkey
- 2 slices cheese (cheddar, swiss, provolone, etc.)
- 1-2 tbsp mayonnaise or mustard (optional)
- Lettuce, tomato, onion (optional toppings)

Instructions:

1. Lay the two slices of bread out on a clean surface. Lightly toast the bread if desired.

2. Spread mayo or mustard on one or both slices, if using.

3. Layer the turkey slices on one slice of bread in an even layer.

4. Top the turkey with the cheese slices.

5. If adding any veggies like lettuce, tomato or onion - add them on top of the cheese.

6. Place the other slice of bread on top to form the sandwich.

7. Press down gently to ensure everything sticks together.

8. If desired, you can grill or toast the assembled sandwich to melt the cheese and warm it through.

9. Cut the sandwich in half diagonally or into quarters.

This turkey and cheese sandwich makes a great lunch, snack or light dinner. It's filling yet simple to make.

You can use any type of sliced deli turkey - oven roasted, smoked, honey roasted, etc. And feel free to mix and match different cheese varieties.

Add extras like bacon, avocado or sprouts to make it even heartier. Just don't overstuff so you can easily pick it up!

46. Chicken Alfredo Pasta

Ingredients:
- 1 cup heavy cream
- 3/4 cup grated parmesan cheese
- 1/4 tsp each salt and pepper
- 2 tbsp chopped fresh parsley
- 8 oz fettuccine or linguine pasta
- 2 boneless, skinless chicken breasts, pounded thin
- 2 tbsp olive oil, divided
- 4 tbsp butter
- 3 cloves garlic, minced

Instructions:

1. Bring a large pot of salted water to a boil. Cook the pasta according to package instructions until al dente. Drain and set aside.

2. Season the chicken breasts with salt and pepper. Heat 1 tbsp olive oil in a skillet over medium-high heat.

3. Cook the chicken for 4-5 minutes per side until no longer pink in the center. Transfer to a plate and cover to keep warm.

4. In the same skillet, heat the remaining 1 tbsp olive oil and 4 tbsp butter over medium heat.

5. Add the minced garlic and cook for 1 minute until fragrant.

6. Pour in the heavy cream and whisk frequently until simmering and slightly thickened, about 2-3 minutes.

7. Remove from heat and whisk in the grated parmesan until fully combined and sauce is smooth.

8. Slice or shred the cooked chicken breasts and add to the alfredo sauce along with the cooked pasta.

9. Toss everything together until the pasta is fully coated in the creamy alfredo sauce. Garnish with chopped parsley and more parmesan if desired. Serve immediately.

This chicken alfredo has such a luscious, velvety sauce coating tender chicken and pasta. It's rich yet so flavorful.

Feel free to add extra seasonings or vegetables like peas, broccoli or sun-dried tomatoes. Fresh cracked pepper on top adds a nice kick. Serve it up with crusty garlic bread or a side salad for a decadent Italian-inspired meal!

47. Soft Baked Potato

Ingredients:
- 4 large russet potatoes
- Olive oil or vegetable oil
- Salt
- Optional toppings: butter, sour cream, chives, bacon bits, shredded cheese

Instructions:

1. Preheat your oven to 400°F (205°C).

2. Scrub the potatoes under running water to remove any dirt or debris. Pat them dry with a paper towel or clean kitchen towel.

3. Using a fork or small knife, prick several holes all over each potato. This allows steam to escape while baking.

4. Rub the potato skins with a thin coating of olive oil or vegetable oil. Then sprinkle generously with salt.

5. Place the potatoes directly on the oven rack in the middle of the oven. Alternatively, you can place them on a baking sheet.

6. Bake for 50-60 minutes, until a knife can easily pierce through the center. Start checking them around 45 minutes.

7. Remove potatoes from oven and make a slit lengthwise across the top. Use an oven mitt as they will be very hot.

8. Give them a gentle squeeze to open up and fluff the insides.

9. Add your favorite toppings like butter, sour cream, chives, bacon bits, shredded cheddar, etc.

The keys are thoroughly pricking holes to vent, rubbing with oil and salt for a crispy skin, and baking at high heat until completely soft in the center.

Baked potatoes make a perfect simple side dish. You can bake them directly on the oven rack or oven-safe baking dish. Enjoy that fluffed potato interior!

48. Buttered Toast

Ingredients:
- 2-4 slices bread (white, whole wheat, etc.)
- Butter, softened at room temperature
- Salt (optional)

Instructions:

1. Toast the bread slices in a toaster or toaster oven to your desired level of doneness. You want them golden brown.

2. Remove the hot toast and immediately transfer it to a plate or cutting board.

3. Take the softened butter and smear or spread it generously over one side of each slice of toast while it's still hot.

4. If desired, you can lightly sprinkle some salt over the buttered toast. The salt enhances the butter flavor.

5. For extra flavor, you can lightly grill or pan fry the buttered toast in a skillet to get a crispy, golden brown outer layer.

6. Cut the buttered toast slices in half diagonally if desired.

7. Serve the buttered toast hot and let any extra butter pool on the plate for dipping the toast edges.

That's all there is to it! The hot toast causes the butter to melt deliciously into all the nooks and crannies.

For a richly flavored twist, try using salted butter or even adding a sprinkle of garlic powder or cinnamon-sugar on top of the buttered toast.

Buttered toast is such a simple but comforting breakfast side. It's also the perfect base for lots of tasty toppings.

49. Baked Ham

Ingredients:
- 1 (5-7 lb) fully cooked bone-in ham
- 1/2 cup brown sugar
- 1/4 cup honey
- 2 tbsp Dijon mustard
- 1 tsp ground cinnamon
- 1/4 tsp ground cloves
- 1/4 cup orange juice or apple cider

Instructions:

1. Remove the ham from its packaging and pat it dry with paper towels. Use a sharp knife to score the ham in a diamond pattern across the top, about 1/4-inch deep.

2. In a small bowl, mix together the brown sugar, honey, Dijon mustard, cinnamon, cloves and orange juice/apple cider until well combined.

3. Place the ham cut-side down in a roasting pan lined with foil (for easy cleanup). Pour 1/2 cup of water into the bottom of the pan.

4. Use a pastry brush or spoon to spread 1/3 of the glaze evenly over the top and sides of the ham.

5. Bake at 325°F for 1 1/2 - 2 hours, basting with the remaining glaze every 30 minutes, until the ham reaches an internal temperature of 140°F.

6. Once glazed and baked, transfer the ham to a cutting board and let it rest for 15 minutes before slicing.

7. Carve the ham by slicing down along the bone in thin slices. Serve with the pan juices spooned over top.

The keys are scoring the ham to allow the glaze to penetrate, basting frequently, and not overcooking. Use a meat thermometer to ensure perfect baking.

This baked ham has a beautifully caramelized, sweet and savory glaze with warm spices. It's an easy but show-stopping holiday centerpiece!

50. Pudding Cups

Ingredients:
- 2 cups milk
- 1 (3.4 oz) package instant pudding mix (chocolate, vanilla, etc.)
- Whipped cream or sprinkles for topping (optional)

Instructions:

1. In a medium bowl, whisk together the 2 cups of milk and the package of instant pudding mix. Whisk vigorously for 2 minutes until the pudding starts to thicken.

2. Pour the pudding mixture evenly into 4-6 small cups, ramekins or pudding cups. Cover with plastic wrap.

3. Refrigerate the pudding cups for at least 2 hours, until completely set. The pudding will continue to thicken as it chills.

4. Once set, remove the plastic wrap. Top each pudding cup with a dollop of whipped cream or sprinkle with toppings of your choice like crushed cookies or chocolate shavings, if desired.

5. Serve the pudding cups chilled. They will keep refrigerated for 3-4 days.

That's it! Instant pudding makes an easy, creamy, nostalgic dessert or snack.

You can use any flavor of instant pudding mix like chocolate, vanilla, butterscotch or even pistachio. The mix-ins and toppings are customizable.

Try layering crushed cookies or graham crackers in the cups before chilling. Or fold in mini chocolate chips, sprinkles or crushed candy right into the pudding before letting it set.

These portable pudding cups satisfy any sweet craving easily! They're rich, creamy and perfect for kids and adults alike.

51. Milk-based Smoothies

1. Classic Strawberry Smoothie
- 1 cup milk (dairy or non-dairy)
- 1 cup frozen strawberries
- 1 banana
- 2 tbsp honey or maple syrup
- 1/2 tsp vanilla extract

2. Tropical Mango Smoothie
- 1 cup milk
- 1 cup frozen mango chunks
- 1/2 banana
- 1/2 cup pineapple chunks
- 1 tbsp honey
- 1/4 tsp ground ginger (optional)

3. Peanut Butter Banana Smoothie
- 1 cup milk
- 1 banana
- 2 tbsp peanut butter
- 1 tbsp honey
- 1/4 tsp cinnamon
- Pinch of nutmeg

4. Green Machine Smoothie
- 1 cup milk
- 1 cup spinach or kale
- 1 banana
- 1/2 cup frozen pineapple chunks
- 1 tbsp honey or agave nectar

5. Chocolate Peanut Butter Smoothie
- 1 cup milk
- 1 banana
- 2 tbsp peanut butter
- 2 tbsp cocoa powder
- 1 tbsp honey
- 1/4 tsp vanilla extract

Instructions:

1. Add all ingredients to a blender and blend until smooth.

2. Adjust sweetness or thickness by adding more milk or honey/syrup as desired.

3. Pour into glasses and enjoy immediately.

You can experiment with different fruits, nut butters, spices, and mix-ins to create endless flavor variations. Milk-based smoothies are a great way to pack in nutrients and make a satisfying snack or light meal.

52. Creamy Mushroom Soup

Ingredients:
- 1/2 cup (115g) unsalted butter
- 1 pound (450g) fresh mushrooms, sliced (cremini, button, or a mix)
- 1 medium onion, diced
- 3 cloves garlic, minced
- 1/4 cup (30g) all-purpose flour
- 4 cups (960ml) chicken or vegetable broth
- 1 cup (240ml) milk
- 1/2 cup (120ml) heavy cream
- 1 tsp dried thyme
- Salt and pepper to taste
- Chopped fresh parsley for garnish

Instructions:

1. In a large pot or dutch oven, melt the butter over medium-high heat. Add the sliced mushrooms and sauté for 5-7 minutes until they start to brown.

2. Add the diced onion and minced garlic. Cook for 2 more minutes until fragrant.

3. Sprinkle the flour over the mushroom mixture and stir to coat everything well. Cook for 1 minute.

4. Gradually pour in the broth while stirring constantly to prevent lumps.

5. Add the milk, cream, thyme, and season with salt and pepper to taste.

6. Bring the soup to a simmer and let it cook for 10-15 minutes, stirring frequently, until it thickens to your desired consistency.

7. Taste and adjust seasonings as needed, adding more salt, pepper or thyme.

8. Remove from heat and optionally use an immersion blender to partially puree some of the mushrooms for a creamier texture (or leave it chunky).

9. Serve the mushroom soup hot, garnished with chopped parsley if desired.

You can make this vegetarian by using vegetable broth. For an extra rich soup, substitute part of the milk for additional cream. The mushrooms give such a savory, umami flavor to this satisfying creamy soup.

53. Rice Pudding with Cinnamon

Ingredients:
- 1/2 cup (100g) white rice (short or long grain)
- 3 cups (720ml) milk
- 1/3 cup (65g) white sugar
- 1/4 tsp salt
- 1 egg, beaten
- 2 tbsp unsalted butter
- 1 tsp vanilla extract
- 1/2 tsp ground cinnamon, plus more for dusting
- 1/4 cup (35g) raisins (optional)

Instructions:

1. In a large saucepan, combine the rice, milk, sugar and salt. Bring to a simmer over medium heat, stirring occasionally.

2. Once simmering, reduce heat to low and cook uncovered for 25-30 minutes, stirring frequently, until the rice is very soft and the mixture is thickened.

3. Remove from heat and let cool slightly. Temper the beaten egg by whisking in a few spoonfuls of the hot rice mixture to slowly raise the temperature.

4. Then whisk the egg into the saucepan with the rice pudding. Return to low heat and cook for 2-3 more minutes, stirring constantly, until thickened slightly more.

5. Remove from heat and stir in the butter, vanilla, 1/2 tsp cinnamon, and raisins if using.

6. Transfer the rice pudding to a bowl or individual ramekins and let cool completely. Refrigerate for at least 2 hours before serving chilled or at room temperature.

7. Before serving, dust the tops with additional ground cinnamon.

This creamy, sweet, and cinnamon-spiced rice pudding makes a wonderfully comforting dessert or snack. For a richer pudding, use half milk and half cream. You can also top it with whipped cream, nuts, or other desired toppings.

54. Baked Salmon Fillet

Ingredients:
- 1 lb (450g) salmon fillet, skin on or off
- 2 tbsp olive oil or melted butter
- 1 tbsp lemon juice
- 2 cloves garlic, minced
- 1 tsp dried dill or 1 tbsp fresh dill, chopped
- Salt and pepper to taste
- Lemon wedges for serving

Instructions:

1. Preheat your oven to 400°F (205°C). Line a baking sheet with foil or parchment paper.

2. Pat the salmon fillet dry with paper towels and place it skin-side down on the prepared baking sheet.

3. In a small bowl, whisk together the olive oil/melted butter, lemon juice, minced garlic, dill, salt and pepper.

4. Brush or spoon the olive oil/butter mixture evenly over the top of the salmon fillet.

5. Bake for 12-15 minutes per inch of thickness, until the salmon flakes easily with a fork in the thickest part. Do not overcook.

6. Optional - For crispier salmon skin, bake for 3-4 minutes under the broiler after baking.

7. Remove from oven and let rest for 5 minutes. The salmon will continue cooking from the residual heat.

8. Transfer salmon to a platter and serve warm with lemon wedges to squeeze over top.

You can customize this by using different herbs like parsley, thyme or rosemary instead of dill. Baking salmon in foil packets with veggies and seasonings is also a great option. Let the thickness of your fillet guide the cooking time for perfect, flaky baked salmon every time.

55. Plain Waffles

Ingredients:
- 2 cups (250g) all-purpose flour
- 1 tbsp (12g) white sugar
- 1 tsp baking powder
- 1/2 tsp baking soda
- 1/2 tsp salt
- 1 3/4 cups (420ml) milk
- 1/3 cup (80ml) vegetable oil or melted butter
- 1 egg
- 1 tsp vanilla extract

Instructions:

1. In a large bowl, whisk together the flour, sugar, baking powder, baking soda and salt.

2. In a separate bowl, whisk together the milk, vegetable oil/melted butter, egg and vanilla.

3. Pour the milk mixture into the flour mixture and whisk together just until combined (do not overmix).

4. Let the waffle batter rest for 5-10 minutes while preheating your waffle iron.

5. Spray the preheated waffle iron with non-stick cooking spray.

6. Pour batter onto the hot waffle iron in batches, using about 1/2 cup per waffle section.

7. Cook for 3-5 minutes until the waffles are golden brown.

8. Remove waffles from iron and keep warm in a 200°F (95°C) oven until ready to serve.

9. Serve the plain waffles hot with your favorite toppings like butter, syrup, fresh fruit, whipped cream, etc.

For crispier waffles, you can separate the egg and whip the whites until stiff peaks form before folding into the batter. This recipe makes about 8-10 waffles, depending on your iron's size. Enjoy these light, crispy yet fluffy homemade waffles!

56. Lemon Jell-O

Ingredients:
- 1 (3 oz) package lemon flavored gelatin mix (like Jell-O)
- 1 cup boiling water
- 1 cup cold water
- Optional: 1-2 tbsp fresh lemon juice

Instructions:

1. In a medium bowl, empty the package of lemon gelatin mix.

2. Add 1 cup of boiling water to the bowl and stir for 2-3 minutes until the gelatin is completely dissolved.

3. Add 1 cup of cold water and optionally 1-2 tbsp of fresh lemon juice if you want a stronger lemon flavor.

4. Stir until well combined.

5. Pour the liquid gelatin mixture into a mold, individual dessert cups or a baking dish.

6. Refrigerate for at least 4 hours or until fully set.

7. Once set, you can slice the Jell-O into squares or cubes if using a mold or baking dish.

8. Serve chilled and enjoy the tangy, refreshing lemon flavor!

For a fancier presentation, try layering the lemon Jell-O with whipped cream or fresh berries before chilling.

You can also make lemon Jell-O jigglers by pouring the mixture into a lightly greased pan and cutting into fun shapes with cookie cutters after chilling.

This is the perfect easy, refreshing treat, especially during spring and summer. The lemon flavor makes it a zingy, vibrant dessert or snack.

57. Turkey Meatballs

Ingredients:
- 1 lb (450g) ground turkey
- 1 egg
- 1/2 cup (40g) breadcrumbs
- 1/4 cup (25g) grated parmesan cheese
- 1/4 cup (15g) finely chopped parsley
- 1 clove garlic, minced
- 1 tsp dried oregano
- 1/2 tsp salt
- 1/4 tsp black pepper
- 2 tbsp olive oil for frying

For the Sauce (Optional):
- 1 (24oz) jar marinara sauce
- 1/4 cup white wine or chicken broth
- 2 tbsp fresh basil, chopped

Instructions:

1. In a large bowl, mix together the ground turkey, egg, breadcrumbs, parmesan, parsley, garlic, oregano, salt and pepper until well combined.

2. Use your hands to form the mixture into golf ball sized meatballs, about 1-2 inches in size.

3. In a large skillet, heat the olive oil over medium-high heat.

4. Add the meatballs in a single layer and brown them on all sides, about 6-8 minutes total.

5. If making the sauce, remove the meatballs and drain excess fat from the pan.

6. Deglaze the pan with the wine/broth, scraping up any browned bits.

7. Add the marinara sauce and meatballs back to the pan. Simmer for 10 minutes.

8. Remove from heat and stir in the fresh basil.

9. Serve the turkey meatballs over pasta, zucchini noodles, or with crusty bread for dipping in the sauce.

Turkey meatballs make a leaner, lighter alternative to beef. The parmesan and herbs add great flavor. You can also bake them on a foil-lined tray at 400°F for 15-20 mins if you prefer.

58. Creamy Chicken and Rice Soup

Ingredients:
- 1 tbsp olive oil
- 1 cup diced carrots
- 1 cup diced celery
- 1 cup diced onion
- 3 cloves garlic, minced
- 8 cups chicken broth
- 1 lb boneless, skinless chicken breasts
- 1 cup long grain white rice
- 1/2 tsp dried thyme
- Salt and pepper to taste
- 1/2 cup heavy cream or half-and-half
- 2 tbsp chopped fresh parsley

Instructions:
1. In a large pot, heat the olive oil over medium heat. Add the carrots, celery, onion and garlic. Sauté for 5 minutes until vegetables are tender.

2. Pour in the chicken broth and add the chicken breasts. Bring to a boil.

3. Once boiling, reduce heat and simmer for 15-20 minutes until chicken is cooked through.

4. Remove the chicken breasts and shred or chop into bite-size pieces. Set aside.

5. Add the rice, thyme, salt and pepper to the pot of broth and vegetables. Simmer for 15 minutes until rice is cooked.

6. Stir in the heavy cream/half-and-half and the cooked shredded chicken.

7. Allow to heat through for 5 more minutes. Taste and adjust seasoning as needed.

8. Remove soup from heat and stir in the chopped parsley.

9. Serve the creamy chicken and rice soup hot, with crusty bread if desired.

This hearty soup has tender chicken, vegetables and rice in a rich, creamy broth. It's perfect for a cozy meal. You can use rotisserie chicken and pre-cooked rice to save time. Top with extra parsley, cheddar cheese or croutons.

59. Mashed Sweet Potatoes

Ingredients:
- 3 lbs (1.4 kg) sweet potatoes, peeled and cut into chunks
- 1/2 cup (120 ml) milk or unsweetened almond milk
- 4 tbsp (55g) unsalted butter
- 2-3 tbsp brown sugar or maple syrup (optional)
- 1 tsp ground cinnamon
- 1/2 tsp ground nutmeg
- 1/2 tsp salt
- 1/4 tsp black pepper
- Chopped pecans or marshmallows for topping (optional)

Instructions:

1. Place the peeled and cut sweet potatoes in a large pot and cover with cold water by 1 inch. Bring to a boil over high heat.

2. Once boiling, reduce heat to medium and simmer for 15-20 minutes, until the sweet potatoes are very soft when pierced with a fork.

3. Drain the cooked sweet potatoes and return them to the hot pot for 1 minute to evaporate any extra moisture.

4. Add the milk, butter, brown sugar/maple syrup (if using), cinnamon, nutmeg, salt and pepper.

5. Use a potato masher or hand mixer to mash the sweet potatoes until smooth and creamy, with some small lumps remaining if desired.

6. Taste and adjust seasoning if needed, adding more butter, sugar, salt, etc.

7. Transfer the mashed sweet potatoes to a serving bowl and top with chopped pecans or mini marshmallows, if desired.

8. Serve warm as a delicious side dish.

You can make these mashed sweet potatoes ahead and reheat them in the oven before serving. The cinnamon and nutmeg add wonderful warmth and spice. For extra richness, use cream or half-and-half instead of milk.

60. Blueberry Smoothie

Ingredients:
- 1 cup fresh or frozen blueberries
- 1 banana
- 1/2 cup Greek yogurt or regular yogurt
- 1/2 cup milk (dairy, almond, oat etc.)
- 2 tbsp honey or maple syrup (optional)
- 1 tsp vanilla extract
- 1 cup ice cubes

Instructions:

1. Add all the ingredients (blueberries, banana, yogurt, milk, honey/maple syrup if using, vanilla, and ice cubes) to a blender.

2. Blend on high speed for 1-2 minutes until smooth and creamy. Stop to scrape down the sides if needed.

3. If the smoothie is too thick, add a splash more milk to reach your desired consistency.

4. Taste and adjust sweetness if needed by adding more honey/maple syrup.

5. Pour the blueberry smoothie into glasses.

6. Optionally garnish with fresh blueberries, banana slices, granola, chia seeds or coconut flakes on top.

7. Serve immediately when nice and chilled.

This blueberry smoothie makes a nutrient-dense breakfast, snack or dessert. The yogurt provides protein while the blueberries are packed with antioxidants. You can use frozen blueberries for an extra thick and frosty smoothie.

For added greens, throw in a handful of spinach or kale. You can also substitute other fruits like strawberries or mixed berries for the blueberries. Enjoy this easy, healthy blueberry smoothie!

61. Cheese Quesadilla

Ingredients:
- 4 large flour tortillas
- 2 cups shredded cheese (cheddar, monterey jack, or a mix)
- 2 tbsp butter or oil for cooking
- Salsa, sour cream, guacamole for serving (optional)

Instructions:

1. Lay two tortillas on a flat surface and sprinkle 1 cup of shredded cheese evenly over one tortilla.

2. Top with the second tortilla to form a quesadilla sandwich.

3. In a large skillet or griddle over medium heat, melt 1 tbsp of the butter or oil.

4. Place the quesadilla in the skillet and cook for 2-3 minutes per side until the tortilla is lightly browned and the cheese is melted.

5. Use a spatula to carefully flip the quesadilla over to cook the other side.

6. Remove the cooked quesadilla from the skillet and let it rest for a minute.

7. Repeat the process with the remaining tortillas, cheese, and butter/oil to make the second quesadilla.

8. Let the quesadillas cool slightly, then slice into wedges using a pizza cutter or knife.

9. Serve the cheese quesadillas warm with salsa, sour cream, and/or guacamole for dipping.

For extra flavor, you can sauté some onions, peppers, or spinach and add them into the quesadilla before cooking. Cooked chicken, beef or beans also make great quesadilla fillings.

These crispy, cheesy, and delightfully simple quesadillas make a crowd-pleasing snack, appetizer or even a quick meal! Adjust the cheese amounts to your preference.

62. Soft Scrambled Eggs

Ingredients:
- 6 large eggs
- 2 tbsp milk or cream
- 1 tbsp butter
- Salt and pepper to taste

Instructions:

1. Crack the eggs into a medium bowl and beat them lightly with a fork or whisk until the yolks and whites are just combined. Don't overbeat.

2. Pour in the milk or cream and season with a pinch of salt and pepper. Whisk to incorporate.

3. Melt the butter in a non-stick skillet over medium-low heat.

4. Once the butter is melted and the skillet is hot, pour in the egg mixture.

5. Use a silicone spatula to gently push and fold the eggs from the edges into the center as they begin to set.

6. Continue folding the eggs every 10-15 seconds, taking care not to overstir.

7. When the eggs are still quite loose and wet with just a few small curds formed, remove from heat.

8. The residual heat will continue cooking the eggs to perfect softly scrambled consistency as you keep folding them for 30 seconds to 1 minute more.

9. Taste and adjust seasoning with additional salt and pepper if needed.

10. Serve the soft, creamy, gently scrambled eggs immediately while hot.

The keys are cooking over lower heat, folding the eggs constantly but gently, and removing them from heat just before they are fully set. This makes for incredibly soft, custard-like scrambled eggs.

Serve with toast, breakfast potatoes, bacon or other breakfast sides. You can also add cheese, herbs or other mix-ins to the eggs.

63. Chicken and Rice Casserole

Ingredients:
- 3 cups cooked chicken, shredded or diced
- 1 cup uncooked long grain white rice
- 1 (10.5 oz) can condensed cream of mushroom soup
- 1 (10.5 oz) can condensed cream of chicken soup
- 1 cup milk
- 1 cup chicken broth
- 1 cup frozen mixed vegetables
- 1 tsp onion powder
- 1/2 tsp garlic powder
- 1/2 tsp dried thyme
- Salt and pepper to taste
- 1 cup shredded cheddar cheese

Instructions:
1. Preheat oven to 375°F (190°C). Grease a 9x13 inch baking dish.

2. In a large bowl, combine the shredded chicken, uncooked rice, condensed soups, milk, chicken broth, frozen vegetables, onion powder, garlic powder, thyme, salt and pepper.

3. Mix everything together until well incorporated.

4. Transfer the chicken and rice mixture to the prepared baking dish.

5. Cover tightly with aluminum foil and bake for 45 minutes.

6. Remove foil and sprinkle the shredded cheddar cheese evenly over the top.

7. Return to oven, uncovered, and bake for 15-20 minutes more until the rice is fully cooked and cheese is melted.

8. Let stand for 5 minutes before serving.

This easy chicken and rice casserole is warm, comforting and so satisfying! You can use rotisserie chicken to save time. Feel free to add extra veggies or swap the soups/seasonings to customize it. Enjoy this family-friendly one-dish meal.

Some options are subbing cream of celery soup, adding broccoli or mushrooms, using brown rice, or topping with breadcrumbs or potato chips before baking. It's endlessly adaptable!

64. Tuna Salad with Mayo

Ingredients:
- 2 (5 oz) cans tuna, drained
- 1/2 cup mayonnaise
- 1/4 cup diced celery
- 2 tbsp diced onion
- 1 tbsp lemon juice
- 1 tsp Dijon mustard
- 1/4 tsp salt
- 1/4 tsp black pepper
- Lettuce leaves or bread, for serving

Instructions:

1. In a medium bowl, flake and break up the drained tuna with a fork.

2. Add the mayonnaise, diced celery, onion, lemon juice, Dijon mustard, salt, and pepper.

3. Mix everything together until well combined, making sure to coat the tuna evenly with the mayonnaise dressing.

4. Taste and adjust seasoning if needed, adding more mayonnaise for moister tuna salad, or lemon juice for extra tanginess.

5. Cover and refrigerate for 30 minutes to allow flavors to blend.

6. When ready to serve, scoop portions of the chilled tuna salad onto lettuce leaves for lettuce wraps or between two slices of bread for sandwiches.

You can add other mix-ins to your tuna salad like chopped hard boiled eggs, dill or sweet pickle relish, chopped apples or grapes for extra crunch and flavor.

Serve this protein-packed tuna salad for a light lunch, afternoon snack or make sandwiches for picnics and meal preps. The creamy mayo dressing perfectly complements the tuna.

It's an easy, no-cook recipe that comes together in just 10 minutes. Adjust amounts of mayo, lemon, celery etc. to your taste preferences.

65. Banana Bread

Ingredients:
- 1 3/4 cups (220g) all-purpose flour
- 1 tsp baking soda
- 1/4 tsp salt
- 1/2 cup (115g) unsalted butter, softened
- 3/4 cup (165g) brown sugar
- 2 large eggs
- 1 1/2 cups (340g) mashed ripe bananas (about 3-4 medium)
- 1/3 cup (80ml) milk
- 1 tsp vanilla extract
- 1/2 cup (60g) chopped walnuts or pecans (optional)

Instructions:
1. Preheat oven to 350°F (177°C). Grease a 9x5 inch loaf pan and line with parchment paper.

2. In a medium bowl, whisk together the flour, baking soda and salt. Set aside.

3. In a large bowl, beat the softened butter and brown sugar until light and fluffy, 2-3 minutes.

4. Beat in the eggs one at a time, then stir in the mashed bananas, milk and vanilla.

5. Fold the dry ingredients into the wet ingredients until just combined, being careful not to overmix.

6. Fold in the chopped nuts if using.

7. Pour the banana bread batter into the prepared loaf pan and smooth the top.

8. Bake for 55-65 minutes, until a toothpick inserted in the center comes out mostly clean.

9. Allow the banana bread to cool in the pan for 10 minutes, then transfer to a wire rack to cool completely before slicing.

This banana bread has incredible moisture and natural sweetness from the ripe bananas. The brown sugar gives it a richer caramel flavor. Enjoy thick slices warm with a pat of butter or cream cheese spread on top.

For variations, you can add chocolate chips, streusel topping, or swap out the nuts for your favorite add-ins. This is a versatile, freezer-friendly bread that makes a great snack or breakfast treat!

66. Milk Rice Pudding

Ingredients:
- 1 cup rice
- 4 cups milk
- 1/2 cup sugar (adjust to taste)
- 1 teaspoon vanilla extract
- 1/4 teaspoon salt
- Cinnamon powder or nutmeg (optional, for garnish)

Instructions:
1. Rinse the rice under cold water until the water runs clear.

2. In a large saucepan, combine the rice, milk, sugar, vanilla extract, and salt.

3. Bring the mixture to a gentle boil over medium heat, stirring occasionally to prevent the rice from sticking to the bottom of the pan.

4. Once boiling, reduce the heat to low and let the mixture simmer uncovered, stirring occasionally, for about 25-30 minutes, or until the rice is cooked and the pudding has thickened to your desired consistency.

5. Remove the pudding from the heat and let it cool slightly before serving.

6. Serve warm or chilled, garnished with a sprinkle of cinnamon powder or nutmeg if desired.

Enjoy your creamy and comforting Milk Rice Pudding!

67. Cheese Toast

Ingredients:
- 4 slices of bread (white, whole wheat, or your preferred type)
- 1 cup shredded cheese (cheddar, mozzarella, or a blend)
- 2 tablespoons butter, softened
- 1/2 teaspoon garlic powder (optional)
- 1/2 teaspoon dried herbs (like oregano or basil, optional)
- Salt and pepper to taste

Instructions:
1. Preheat your oven to 400°F (200°C) or set your broiler to high.

2. Spread a thin layer of softened butter on one side of each slice of bread.

3. If using garlic powder and dried herbs, mix them into the butter before spreading it on the bread.

4. Place the slices of bread, buttered side up, on a baking sheet.

5. Sprinkle an even layer of shredded cheese on top of each slice.

6. Season with a pinch of salt and pepper.

7. Place the baking sheet in the oven and bake for 8-10 minutes, or until the cheese is melted and bubbly, and the edges of the bread are golden brown.

   - If using the broiler, place the baking sheet under the broiler and broil for 2-4 minutes, watching closely to prevent burning, until the cheese is melted and bubbly.

8. Remove from the oven and let cool slightly before serving.

Enjoy your delicious and easy Cheese Toast!

68. Vanilla Yogurt Parfait

Ingredients:
- 2 cups vanilla yogurt
- 1 cup granola
- 1 cup fresh berries (such as strawberries, blueberries, raspberries, or a mix)
- 2 tablespoons honey or maple syrup (optional)
- Fresh mint leaves for garnish (optional)

Instructions:
1. Gather all your ingredients and have them ready to layer.

2. In a tall glass or parfait cup, start by adding a few spoonfuls of vanilla yogurt to the bottom.

3. Add a layer of granola on top of the yogurt.

4. Add a layer of fresh berries over the granola.

5. Repeat the layers until you reach the top of the glass, ending with a layer of yogurt.

6. Drizzle honey or maple syrup on top, if using.

7. Garnish with a few more berries and a sprig of fresh mint, if desired.

8. Serve immediately and enjoy your delicious and healthy Vanilla Yogurt Parfait!

This parfait makes for a great breakfast, snack, or even a light dessert.

69. Creamy Chicken Pasta

Ingredients:
- 2 cups uncooked pasta (penne, fettuccine, or your favorite type)
- 2 tablespoons olive oil
- 1 pound boneless, skinless chicken breasts, cut into bite-sized pieces
- 3 cloves garlic, minced
- 1 cup heavy cream
- 1/2 cup chicken broth
- 1 cup grated Parmesan cheese
- 1 teaspoon Italian seasoning
- Salt and pepper to taste
- 1 cup spinach leaves (optional)
- Fresh parsley, chopped (for garnish)

Instructions:

1. Cook the pasta according to the package instructions until al dente. Drain and set aside.

2. In a large skillet, heat the olive oil over medium-high heat. Add the chicken pieces and season with salt and pepper. Cook until the chicken is browned and cooked through, about 5-7 minutes. Remove the chicken from the skillet and set aside.

3. In the same skillet, add the minced garlic and cook for about 1 minute until fragrant.

4. Pour in the heavy cream and chicken broth, stirring to combine. Bring the mixture to a simmer.

5. Add the Parmesan cheese and Italian seasoning, stirring until the cheese is melted and the sauce is smooth and creamy.

6. Add the cooked chicken back into the skillet, along with the pasta. Toss to coat everything evenly in the sauce.
   - If using spinach, add it now and stir until it wilts.

7. Taste and adjust the seasoning with more salt and pepper if needed. Garnish with chopped fresh parsley before serving.

70. Poached Chicken Salad

Ingredients:
For Poached Chicken:
- 2 boneless, skinless chicken breasts
- 4 cups chicken broth or water
- 2 cloves garlic, smashed
- 1 teaspoon whole peppercorns
- 1 bay leaf
- Salt, to taste

For Dressing:
- 2 tablespoons olive oil
- 1 tablespoon lemon juice or vinegar
 (apple cider vinegar or white wine vinegar)
- 1 teaspoon Dijon mustard
- Salt and pepper, to taste

For Salad:
- 4 cups mixed salad greens
(lettuce, spinach, arugula, etc.)
- 1 cucumber, sliced
- 1 cup cherry tomatoes, halved
- 1/2 red onion, thinly sliced
- 1 avocado, diced
- 1/4 cup fresh cilantro or parsley,
chopped (optional)

Instructions:
1. In a large pot, combine the chicken breasts, chicken broth or water, smashed garlic cloves, whole peppercorns, bay leaf, and salt. Bring to a gentle simmer over medium heat.

2. Once simmering, reduce the heat to low, cover, and let the chicken poach for about 15-20 minutes, or until cooked through. Make sure the internal temperature of the chicken reaches 165°F (75°C).

3. Once cooked, remove the chicken from the poaching liquid and let it cool slightly. Then, shred or slice the chicken into bite-sized pieces.

4. While the chicken is cooling, prepare the salad ingredients. In a large bowl, combine the mixed salad greens, sliced cucumber, cherry tomatoes, red onion, avocado, and chopped cilantro or parsley.

5. In a small bowl, whisk together the olive oil, lemon juice or vinegar, Dijon mustard, salt, and pepper to make the dressing.

6. Add the shredded or sliced poached chicken to the salad bowl. Drizzle the dressing over the salad and toss gently to coat everything evenly. Serve the poached chicken salad immediately, garnished with additional chopped herbs if desired.

71. Soft Boiled Potatoes

Ingredients:
- 4 medium-sized potatoes (any variety you prefer)
- Salt, to taste
- Optional: Butter, chopped fresh herbs (such as parsley or chives)

Instructions:
1. Start by scrubbing the potatoes under cold running water to remove any dirt.

2. Place the potatoes in a large pot and cover them with cold water. Add a generous pinch of salt to the water.

3. Bring the water to a boil over high heat.

4. Once boiling, reduce the heat to medium-low to maintain a gentle simmer.

5. Cook the potatoes for about 15-20 minutes, depending on their size, until they are tender when pierced with a fork. Keep an eye on them to prevent overcooking.

6. Once the potatoes are cooked, carefully remove them from the pot using a slotted spoon and transfer them to a plate or cutting board.

7. Allow the potatoes to cool slightly before serving.

8. To serve, you can either peel the potatoes if desired or leave the skins on. Serve them whole or cut them into halves or quarters.

9. Optionally, you can add a pat of butter and sprinkle chopped fresh herbs over the soft-boiled potatoes before serving for extra flavor.

Enjoy your soft-boiled potatoes as a tasty and comforting side dish!

72. Buttermilk Pancakes

Ingredients:
- 1 1/2 cups all-purpose flour
- 2 tablespoons granulated sugar
- 1 teaspoon baking powder
- 1/2 teaspoon baking soda
- 1/4 teaspoon salt
- 1 1/4 cups buttermilk
- 1 large egg
- 2 tablespoons unsalted butter, melted
- Butter or oil for cooking
- Maple syrup, berries, or other toppings of your choice

Instructions:

1. In a large mixing bowl, whisk together the flour, sugar, baking powder, baking soda, and salt until well combined.

2. In a separate bowl, whisk together the buttermilk, egg, and melted butter until smooth.

3. Pour the wet ingredients into the dry ingredients and gently stir until just combined. It's okay if the batter is a little lumpy; overmixing can make the pancakes tough.

4. Heat a non-stick skillet or griddle over medium heat and lightly grease with butter or oil.

5. Once the skillet is hot, pour about 1/4 cup of batter onto the skillet for each pancake. Use the back of a spoon to spread the batter into a round shape if needed.

6. Cook the pancakes for 2-3 minutes, or until bubbles start to form on the surface and the edges look set.

7. Carefully flip the pancakes using a spatula and cook for an additional 1-2 minutes, or until golden brown and cooked through.

8. Transfer the cooked pancakes to a plate and cover with a clean kitchen towel to keep warm while you cook the remaining batter.

9. Serve the pancakes warm with maple syrup, fresh berries, or your favorite toppings.

Enjoy your fluffy and delicious Buttermilk Pancakes for a delightful breakfast or brunch!

73. Mashed Cauliflower

Ingredients:
- 1 large head of cauliflower, chopped into florets
- 2 cloves garlic, minced
- 2 tablespoons butter or olive oil
- 1/4 cup grated Parmesan cheese (optional)
- Salt and pepper, to taste
- Chopped fresh parsley or chives, for garnish (optional)

Instructions:

1. Bring a large pot of salted water to a boil. Add the cauliflower florets and minced garlic to the boiling water and cook for about 10-12 minutes, or until the cauliflower is very tender.

2. Drain the cooked cauliflower and garlic well, then transfer them to a large bowl.

3. Using a potato masher or fork, mash the cauliflower and garlic until smooth. You can also use a food processor for a smoother consistency.

4. Add the butter or olive oil to the mashed cauliflower and mix until well combined. Stir in the grated Parmesan cheese if using.

5. Season the mashed cauliflower with salt and pepper to taste. Adjust the seasoning as needed.

6. Transfer the mashed cauliflower to a serving dish and garnish with chopped fresh parsley or chives if desired.

7. Serve the mashed cauliflower hot as a delicious and nutritious side dish.

Enjoy your creamy and flavorful Mashed Cauliflower!

74. Chicken Broccoli Casserole

Ingredients:
- 2 cups cooked chicken, diced or shredded
- 2 cups broccoli florets, blanched
- 1 1/2 cups cooked rice
- 1 can (10.5 oz) condensed cream of chicken soup
- 1 cup sour cream
- 1 cup shredded cheddar cheese
- 1/2 cup grated Parmesan cheese
- 1/2 cup milk
- 2 cloves garlic, minced
- 1 teaspoon onion powder
- 1/2 teaspoon dried thyme
- Salt and pepper, to taste
- 1 cup breadcrumbs
- 2 tablespoons melted butter

Instructions:
1. Preheat your oven to 350°F (175°C). Grease a 9x13-inch baking dish and set aside.

2. In a large mixing bowl, combine the cooked chicken, blanched broccoli florets, cooked rice, condensed cream of chicken soup, sour cream, shredded cheddar cheese, grated Parmesan cheese, milk, minced garlic, onion powder, dried thyme, salt, and pepper. Mix until well combined.

3. Spread the mixture evenly into the prepared baking dish.

4. In a small bowl, combine the breadcrumbs and melted butter. Sprinkle the breadcrumb mixture evenly over the top of the casserole.

5. Cover the baking dish with aluminum foil and bake in the preheated oven for 25 minutes.

6. After 25 minutes, remove the foil and continue baking for an additional 10-15 minutes, or until the casserole is bubbly and the breadcrumbs are golden brown.

7. Remove from the oven and let it cool for a few minutes before serving.

8. Serve the chicken broccoli casserole hot as a delicious and comforting meal.

Enjoy your hearty and flavorful Chicken Broccoli Casserole!

75. Potato Leek Soup

Ingredients:
- 3 leeks, white and light green parts only, sliced
- 3 large potatoes, peeled and diced
- 4 cups vegetable or chicken broth
- 1 cup heavy cream or milk
- 2 tablespoons butter
- Salt and pepper, to taste
- Chopped fresh chives or parsley, for garnish (optional)

Instructions:

1. In a large pot or Dutch oven, melt the butter over medium heat. Add the sliced leeks and cook, stirring occasionally, until softened, about 5-7 minutes.

2. Add the diced potatoes to the pot and pour in the vegetable or chicken broth. Bring the mixture to a simmer.

3. Reduce the heat to low, cover, and let the soup simmer for about 15-20 minutes, or until the potatoes are tender.

4. Using an immersion blender or regular blender, blend the soup until smooth and creamy. Be careful when blending hot liquids.

5. Stir in the heavy cream or milk and season the soup with salt and pepper to taste. Adjust the seasoning as needed.

6. Continue to simmer the soup for a few more minutes to heat through.

7. Serve the potato leek soup hot, garnished with chopped fresh chives or parsley if desired.

8. Enjoy your creamy and flavorful Potato Leek Soup as a comforting meal!

This soup pairs well with crusty bread or a simple salad for a satisfying lunch or dinner.

76. Mashed Turnips

Ingredients:
- 2 pounds turnips, peeled and diced
- 2 cloves garlic, minced (optional)
- 2 tablespoons butter
- 1/4 cup heavy cream or milk
- Salt and pepper, to taste
- Chopped fresh parsley or chives, for garnish (optional)

Instructions:

1. Place the diced turnips in a large pot and cover them with water. Add a generous pinch of salt to the water.

2. Bring the water to a boil over medium-high heat. Reduce the heat to medium-low and let the turnips simmer for about 15-20 minutes, or until they are tender when pierced with a fork.

3. Drain the cooked turnips well and transfer them to a large mixing bowl.

4. Using a potato masher or fork, mash the turnips until they reach your desired consistency. You can also use a food processor for a smoother texture.

5. In a small saucepan, melt the butter over low heat. Add the minced garlic, if using, and cook for 1-2 minutes until fragrant.

6. Pour the melted butter (with garlic) over the mashed turnips.

7. Add the heavy cream or milk to the mashed turnips and stir until well combined. You can adjust the amount of cream or milk to achieve your preferred consistency.

8. Season the mashed turnips with salt and pepper to taste. Adjust the seasoning as needed.

9. Transfer the mashed turnips to a serving dish and garnish with chopped fresh parsley or chives, if desired.

10. Serve the mashed turnips hot as a delicious and nutritious side dish.

Enjoy your creamy and flavorful Mashed Turnips!

77. Creamy Spinach Dip

Ingredients:
- 1 (10 oz) package frozen chopped spinach, thawed and drained
- 1 cup sour cream
- 1 cup mayonnaise
- 1 packet (about 1 oz) dry vegetable soup mix (such as onion soup mix)
- 1 cup shredded mozzarella cheese
- 1/2 cup grated Parmesan cheese
- 1 teaspoon garlic powder
- Salt and pepper, to taste
- Optional: Chopped green onions or chives, for garnish

Instructions:
1. Preheat your oven to 350°F (175°C).

2. In a large mixing bowl, combine the drained spinach, sour cream, mayonnaise, dry vegetable soup mix, shredded mozzarella cheese, grated Parmesan cheese, garlic powder, salt, and pepper. Mix until well combined.

3. Transfer the mixture to a baking dish or oven-safe skillet, spreading it out evenly.

4. Bake in the preheated oven for 25-30 minutes, or until the dip is hot and bubbly and the cheese is melted and golden brown on top.

5. Remove the dip from the oven and let it cool for a few minutes before serving.

6. If desired, garnish the creamy spinach dip with chopped green onions or chives before serving.

7. Serve the dip warm with tortilla chips, crackers, sliced baguette, or vegetable sticks for dipping.

Enjoy your delicious and creamy Spinach Dip as a crowd-pleasing appetizer!

78. Turkey Bacon Omelette

Ingredients:
- 2 large eggs
- 2 slices turkey bacon, chopped
- 1/4 cup shredded cheddar cheese
- 1 tablespoon chopped fresh parsley or chives (optional)
- Salt and pepper, to taste
- 1 teaspoon butter or cooking oil

Instructions:

1. In a small bowl, beat the eggs until well combined. Season with salt and pepper to taste. Set aside.

2. In a non-stick skillet, cook the chopped turkey bacon over medium heat until crispy, about 5-7 minutes. Remove the bacon from the skillet and set aside.

3. Wipe out any excess grease from the skillet, leaving a thin coating.

4. Return the skillet to the heat and add the butter or cooking oil, swirling to coat the bottom of the skillet evenly.

5. Pour the beaten eggs into the skillet, tilting the skillet to spread the eggs out evenly.

6. Cook the eggs for 1-2 minutes, or until the edges begin to set.

7. Sprinkle the cooked turkey bacon and shredded cheddar cheese evenly over one half of the omelette.

8. Using a spatula, carefully fold the other half of the omelette over the filling.

9. Cook the omelette for another 1-2 minutes, or until the cheese is melted and the eggs are cooked through.

10. Slide the omelette onto a plate and sprinkle with chopped fresh parsley or chives, if desired.

11. Serve the Turkey Bacon Omelette hot, with toast or a side salad if desired.

Enjoy your flavorful and satisfying Turkey Bacon Omelette for breakfast or brunch!

79. Soft Cheese Tacos

Ingredients:
- 8 small flour or corn tortillas
- 1 cup shredded cheese (such as cheddar, Monterey Jack, or a Mexican blend)
- Optional toppings: diced tomatoes, sliced avocado, chopped lettuce, salsa, sour cream, sliced jalapeños, chopped cilantro, lime wedges, etc.

Instructions:

1. Warm the tortillas: You can heat them in a skillet over medium heat for about 30 seconds on each side until warm and pliable, or wrap them in a damp paper towel and microwave them for about 20-30 seconds.

2. Assemble the tacos: Place a spoonful of shredded cheese in the center of each tortilla.

3. Add your desired toppings: Get creative! You can add diced tomatoes, sliced avocado, chopped lettuce, salsa, sour cream, sliced jalapeños, chopped cilantro, a squeeze of lime juice, or any other toppings you like.

4. Serve immediately: Enjoy your soft cheese tacos while they're warm and the cheese is melted.

These soft cheese tacos are customizable, so feel free to get creative and add your favorite ingredients to make them your own!

80. Potato Soup

Ingredients:

- 4 medium potatoes, peeled and diced
- 1 onion, diced
- 2 cloves garlic, minced
- 4 cups vegetable or chicken broth
- 1 cup milk or cream
- 2 tablespoons butter
- 2 tablespoons all-purpose flour
- Salt and pepper, to taste
- Optional toppings: shredded cheese, chopped green onions or chives, crispy bacon bits, sour cream, etc.

Instructions:

1. In a large pot or Dutch oven, melt the butter over medium heat. Add the diced onion and garlic, and cook until softened and fragrant, about 5 minutes.

2. Add the diced potatoes to the pot, along with the vegetable or chicken broth. Bring the mixture to a boil, then reduce the heat to low and let it simmer for about 15-20 minutes, or until the potatoes are tender.

3. In a separate small bowl, whisk together the milk or cream and flour until smooth. Pour the mixture into the pot, stirring constantly.

4. Continue to cook the soup for another 5 minutes, or until it thickens slightly.

5. Using an immersion blender or regular blender, blend the soup until smooth. If you prefer a chunkier soup, you can skip this step or blend only part of the soup.

6. Season the soup with salt and pepper to taste. Adjust the seasoning as needed.

7. Serve the potato soup hot, garnished with your choice of toppings such as shredded cheese, chopped green onions or chives, crispy bacon bits, sour cream, etc.

Enjoy your creamy and delicious Potato Soup as a comforting meal!

81. Grilled Salmon Salad

Ingredients:

For Grilled Salmon:
- 2 salmon fillets (about 6 ounces each)
- 1 tablespoon olive oil
- Salt and pepper, to taste
- Lemon wedges, for serving (optional)

For Dressing:
- 2 tablespoons olive oil
- 1 tablespoon lemon juice
- 1 teaspoon Dijon mustard
- 1 teaspoon honey or
maple syrup (optional)
- Salt and pepper, to taste

For Salad:
- 6 cups mixed salad greens
(such as lettuce, spinach,
arugula, etc.)
- 1 cucumber, sliced
- 1 cup cherry tomatoes, halved
- 1/4 red onion, thinly sliced
- 1 avocado, sliced
- 1/4 cup sliced almonds or
chopped walnuts (optional)
- 2 tablespoons chopped fresh
herbs (such as dill, parsley, or
cilantro)

Instructions:

1. Preheat your grill to medium-high heat.

2. Brush the salmon fillets with olive oil and season with salt and pepper.

3. Place the salmon fillets on the grill, skin-side down, and cook for about 4-5 minutes per side, or until the salmon is cooked through and easily flakes with a fork. Cooking time may vary depending on the thickness of the fillets.

4. While the salmon is grilling, prepare the salad ingredients. In a large bowl, combine the mixed salad greens, sliced cucumber, cherry tomatoes, red onion, avocado, sliced almonds or chopped walnuts (if using), and chopped fresh herbs.

5. In a small bowl, whisk together the olive oil, lemon juice, Dijon mustard, honey or maple syrup (if using), salt, and pepper to make the dressing.

6. Once the salmon is cooked, remove it from the grill and let it cool slightly. Use a fork to flake the salmon into bite-sized pieces.

7. Add the grilled salmon to the salad bowl.

8. Drizzle the dressing over the salad and toss gently to coat everything evenly.

9. Serve the grilled salmon salad immediately, with lemon wedges on the side for squeezing over the salmon if desired.

82. Rice Pudding with Berries

Ingredients:
- 1 cup short-grain rice (like Arborio)
- 4 cups milk (whole milk preferred for creaminess)
- 1/2 cup sugar
- 1 teaspoon vanilla extract
- 1/4 teaspoon salt
- 1 cup mixed berries (such as strawberries, blueberries, raspberries, or blackberries)
- Optional: ground cinnamon or nutmeg for garnish

Instructions:

1. Rinse the rice under cold water until the water runs clear. This helps remove excess starch and prevents the pudding from becoming too sticky.

2. In a large saucepan, combine the rice, milk, sugar, vanilla extract, and salt. Stir to mix well.

3. Bring the mixture to a gentle boil over medium heat, stirring frequently to prevent the rice from sticking to the bottom of the pan.

4. Once it reaches a boil, reduce the heat to low and let it simmer gently. Continue to cook for about 30-40 minutes, stirring occasionally, until the rice is tender and the mixture has thickened to a creamy consistency. If the pudding becomes too thick, you can add a little more milk to reach your desired consistency.

5. While the rice pudding is cooking, prepare the berries. Wash and hull the strawberries if using them, and cut them into bite-sized pieces. If using other berries, wash them and set aside.

6. Once the rice pudding is cooked, remove it from the heat and let it cool slightly. The pudding will continue to thicken as it cools.

7. Serve the rice pudding warm or chilled, topped with the mixed berries. You can also sprinkle a bit of ground cinnamon or nutmeg on top for extra flavor.

8. If you prefer, you can gently fold some of the berries into the pudding before serving, reserving a few for garnish on top.

Enjoy your creamy and delicious Rice Pudding with Berries!

83. Chicken Noodle Soup (strained)

Ingredients:
- 2 boneless, skinless chicken breasts
- 8 cups chicken broth
- 2 carrots, peeled and sliced
- 2 celery stalks, sliced
- 1 onion, diced
- 2 cloves garlic, minced
- 1 bay leaf
- 1 teaspoon dried thyme
- Salt and pepper, to taste
- 6 ounces egg noodles
- Chopped fresh parsley, for garnish (optional)

Instructions:
1. In a large pot, combine the chicken breasts, chicken broth, carrots, celery, onion, garlic, bay leaf, dried thyme, salt, and pepper.

2. Bring the mixture to a boil over medium-high heat, then reduce the heat to low and let it simmer, partially covered, for about 20-25 minutes, or until the chicken is cooked through and tender.

3. Remove the chicken breasts from the pot and transfer them to a cutting board. Use two forks to shred the chicken into bite-sized pieces.

4. Meanwhile, strain the soup through a fine mesh sieve or cheesecloth-lined colander into another large pot or bowl. Discard the solids (carrots, celery, onion, etc.) or reserve them for another use if desired.

5. Return the strained broth to the pot and bring it back to a simmer over medium heat.

6. Add the shredded chicken back into the pot along with the egg noodles. Let the soup simmer for an additional 8-10 minutes, or until the noodles are cooked through and tender.

7. Taste the soup and adjust the seasoning with more salt and pepper if needed.

8. Ladle the strained Chicken Noodle Soup into bowls and garnish with chopped fresh parsley, if desired.

Enjoy your comforting and soothing Chicken Noodle Soup!

84. Cheese Ravioli

Ingredients:
- 1 package (about 12-16 ounces) cheese ravioli (fresh or frozen)
- 2 tablespoons butter
- 2 cloves garlic, minced
- 1/4 cup grated Parmesan cheese
- Salt and pepper, to taste
- Chopped fresh parsley or basil, for garnish (optional)

Instructions:

1. Cook the cheese ravioli according to the package instructions. If using frozen ravioli, boil them in a pot of salted water for about 3-4 minutes until they float to the surface. If using fresh ravioli, follow the recommended cooking time provided on the package.

2. While the ravioli is cooking, melt the butter in a large skillet over medium heat.

3. Add the minced garlic to the skillet and cook for 1-2 minutes, or until fragrant.

4. Once the ravioli is cooked, use a slotted spoon to transfer them directly from the pot to the skillet with the garlic butter. Toss gently to coat the ravioli in the butter and garlic.

5. Sprinkle the grated Parmesan cheese over the ravioli and continue to toss until the cheese is melted and the ravioli are evenly coated.

6. Season with salt and pepper to taste. Be mindful of the saltiness of the Parmesan cheese before adding too much salt.

7. Remove the skillet from the heat and transfer the cheese ravioli to serving plates.

8. Garnish with chopped fresh parsley or basil, if desired.

9. Serve the cheese ravioli hot as a delicious and satisfying meal.

Enjoy your quick and tasty Cheese Ravioli!

85. Creamy Zucchini Soup

Ingredients:
- 2 tablespoons olive oil or butter
- 1 onion, chopped
- 2 cloves garlic, minced
- 4 medium zucchinis, chopped
- 4 cups vegetable or chicken broth
- 1/2 cup heavy cream or milk
- Salt and pepper, to taste
- Fresh herbs (such as basil, parsley, or dill) for garnish (optional)
- Optional: 1/4 cup grated Parmesan cheese for extra flavor

Instructions:

1. In a large pot, heat the olive oil or butter over medium heat. Add the chopped onion and cook until it becomes translucent, about 5 minutes.

2. Add the minced garlic and cook for another 1-2 minutes, until fragrant.

3. Add the chopped zucchinis to the pot and stir to combine with the onions and garlic. Cook for about 5-7 minutes, allowing the zucchinis to soften slightly.

4. Pour in the vegetable or chicken broth and bring the mixture to a boil. Once boiling, reduce the heat to low and let it simmer for about 15-20 minutes, or until the zucchinis are tender.

5. Using an immersion blender, blend the soup until smooth and creamy. If you don't have an immersion blender, you can carefully transfer the soup in batches to a regular blender and blend until smooth. Be cautious with hot liquids.

6. Return the blended soup to the pot (if using a regular blender) and stir in the heavy cream or milk. If you're using Parmesan cheese, add it now and stir until melted and well incorporated.

7. Season the soup with salt and pepper to taste. Adjust the seasoning as needed.

8. Let the soup simmer for another 5 minutes to heat through.

9. Serve the creamy zucchini soup hot, garnished with fresh herbs if desired.

Enjoy your delicious and creamy Zucchini Soup!

86. Baked Chicken Thighs

Ingredients:
- 6 bone-in, skin-on chicken thighs
- 2 tablespoons olive oil
- 3 cloves garlic, minced
- 1 teaspoon dried thyme
- 1 teaspoon dried rosemary
- 1 teaspoon paprika
- Salt and pepper, to taste
- Optional: fresh lemon slices and chopped fresh parsley for garnish

Instructions:
1. Preheat your oven to 400°F (200°C).

2. Pat the chicken thighs dry with paper towels. This helps to ensure a crispy skin.

3. In a small bowl, mix together the olive oil, minced garlic, dried thyme, dried rosemary, paprika, salt, and pepper.

4. Rub the olive oil mixture evenly over the chicken thighs, making sure to get some of the mixture under the skin for extra flavor.

5. Place the chicken thighs in a single layer on a baking sheet or in a baking dish, skin side up.

6. If using, arrange the fresh lemon slices around the chicken thighs for added flavor.

7. Bake in the preheated oven for 35-45 minutes, or until the chicken thighs reach an internal temperature of 165°F (75°C) and the skin is crispy and golden brown.

8. Remove the chicken thighs from the oven and let them rest for a few minutes before serving.

9. Garnish with chopped fresh parsley if desired.

10. Serve the baked chicken thighs hot, with your choice of sides such as roasted vegetables, mashed potatoes, or a fresh salad.

Enjoy your juicy and flavorful Baked Chicken Thighs!

87. Turkey and Rice Stew

Ingredients:
- 1 lb turkey breast, diced (or use leftover cooked turkey)
- 2 tablespoons olive oil
- 1 onion, chopped
- 2 cloves garlic, minced
- 2 carrots, peeled and sliced
- 2 celery stalks, sliced
- 1 cup uncooked rice (white or brown)
- 6 cups chicken or turkey broth
- 1 teaspoon dried thyme
- 1 teaspoon dried rosemary
- 1 bay leaf
- Salt and pepper, to taste
- 1 cup frozen peas (optional)
- 1/4 cup chopped fresh parsley, for garnish

Instructions:

1. In a large pot or Dutch oven, heat the olive oil over medium heat. Add the diced turkey breast and cook until browned, about 5-7 minutes. If using leftover cooked turkey, add it later in the cooking process.

2. Add the chopped onion, minced garlic, carrots, and celery to the pot. Cook, stirring occasionally, until the vegetables are softened, about 5 minutes.

3. Stir in the uncooked rice, dried thyme, dried rosemary, bay leaf, salt, and pepper. Cook for another 1-2 minutes, allowing the rice to lightly toast.

4. Pour in the chicken or turkey broth and bring the mixture to a boil.

5. Reduce the heat to low, cover the pot, and let the stew simmer for about 20-25 minutes, or until the rice is tender and the flavors have melded together. If using leftover cooked turkey, add it now and allow it to heat through.

6. If you're adding frozen peas, stir them into the stew during the last 5 minutes of cooking.

7. Remove the bay leaf and discard.

8. Taste the stew and adjust the seasoning with more salt and pepper if needed. Serve the turkey and rice stew hot, garnished with chopped fresh parsley.

88. Creamy Corn Soup

Ingredients:
- 2 tablespoons butter
- 1 onion, chopped
- 2 cloves garlic, minced
- 4 cups corn kernels (fresh, frozen, or canned, drained)
- 4 cups vegetable or chicken broth
- 1 cup heavy cream or milk
- 1 teaspoon dried thyme
- Salt and pepper, to taste
- Optional: 1/4 teaspoon smoked paprika or cayenne pepper for a bit of heat
- Chopped fresh parsley or chives, for garnish

Instructions:
1. In a large pot, melt the butter over medium heat. Add the chopped onion and cook until it becomes translucent, about 5 minutes.

2. Add the minced garlic and cook for another 1-2 minutes, until fragrant.

3. Stir in the corn kernels, vegetable or chicken broth, and dried thyme. Bring the mixture to a boil.

4. Reduce the heat to low and let it simmer for about 15-20 minutes, allowing the flavors to meld together.

5. Using an immersion blender, blend the soup until smooth and creamy. If you prefer a chunkier texture, blend only part of the soup. If you don't have an immersion blender, carefully transfer the soup in batches to a regular blender and blend until smooth. Be cautious with hot liquids.

6. Return the blended soup to the pot (if using a regular blender) and stir in the heavy cream or milk. If you're adding smoked paprika or cayenne pepper, stir it in now.

7. Season the soup with salt and pepper to taste. Adjust the seasoning as needed.

8. Let the soup simmer for another 5 minutes to heat through.

9. Serve the creamy corn soup hot, garnished with chopped fresh parsley or chives.

Enjoy your delicious and comforting Creamy Corn Soup!

89. Macaroni in Cream Sauce

Ingredients:
- 8 ounces macaroni (or any pasta of your choice)
- 2 tablespoons butter
- 2 tablespoons all-purpose flour
- 2 cups milk (whole milk preferred for creaminess)
- 1 cup grated Parmesan cheese (or any cheese of your choice, such as cheddar or Gruyère)
- Salt and pepper, to taste
- Pinch of ground nutmeg (optional)
- Chopped fresh parsley, for garnish (optional)

Instructions:

1. Cook the macaroni according to the package instructions until al dente. Drain and set aside.

2. In a large saucepan, melt the butter over medium heat. Once melted, add the flour and whisk continuously to form a roux. Cook for about 1-2 minutes until the roux is golden and has a slightly nutty aroma.

3. Gradually add the milk to the roux, whisking constantly to avoid lumps. Continue to cook, stirring frequently, until the sauce thickens and starts to simmer, about 5-7 minutes.

4. Reduce the heat to low and stir in the grated Parmesan cheese until it melts and the sauce is smooth. If using, add a pinch of ground nutmeg for extra flavor.

5. Season the cream sauce with salt and pepper to taste. Adjust the seasoning as needed.

6. Add the cooked macaroni to the cream sauce, stirring to coat the pasta evenly with the sauce.

7. Cook for an additional 2-3 minutes, allowing the pasta to absorb some of the sauce and heat through.

8. Serve the macaroni in cream sauce hot, garnished with chopped fresh parsley if desired.

Enjoy your creamy and delicious Macaroni in Cream Sauce!

90. Lemon Gelatin Cups

Ingredients:
- 1 package (3 ounces) lemon-flavored gelatin
- 1 cup boiling water
- 1 cup cold water
- 1 tablespoon lemon juice (optional, for extra lemon flavor)
- Whipped cream, for topping (optional)
- Lemon zest or fresh mint leaves, for garnish (optional)

Instructions:

1. In a medium bowl, dissolve the lemon gelatin in the boiling water, stirring for about 2 minutes until completely dissolved.

2. Stir in the cold water and lemon juice (if using). Mix well.

3. Pour the gelatin mixture into individual serving cups or bowls.

4. Refrigerate the gelatin cups for at least 4 hours, or until fully set.

5. Once set, you can top the lemon gelatin cups with a dollop of whipped cream if desired.

6. Garnish with lemon zest or fresh mint leaves for an extra touch of flavor and presentation.

7. Serve chilled.

Enjoy your refreshing Lemon Gelatin Cups!

91. Baked Pork Chops

Ingredients:
- 4 bone-in or boneless pork chops (about 1-inch thick)
- 2 tablespoons olive oil
- 2 cloves garlic, minced
- 1 teaspoon dried thyme
- 1 teaspoon dried rosemary
- 1 teaspoon paprika
- Salt and pepper, to taste
- Optional: lemon wedges and fresh parsley for garnish

Instructions:

1. Preheat your oven to 400°F (200°C).

2. Pat the pork chops dry with paper towels. This helps them to sear properly and get a nice crust.

3. In a small bowl, mix together the olive oil, minced garlic, dried thyme, dried rosemary, paprika, salt, and pepper.

4. Rub the seasoning mixture evenly over both sides of each pork chop.

5. Heat a large oven-safe skillet over medium-high heat. Once hot, add a little more olive oil if needed, and sear the pork chops for about 2-3 minutes on each side until they are golden brown.

6. Transfer the skillet with the pork chops to the preheated oven. If you don't have an oven-safe skillet, you can transfer the pork chops to a baking dish.

7. Bake the pork chops in the oven for about 15-20 minutes, or until the internal temperature reaches 145°F (63°C) for medium or 160°F (71°C) for well done. The baking time will depend on the thickness of the pork chops.

8. Remove the pork chops from the oven and let them rest for 5 minutes before serving. This allows the juices to redistribute, making the pork chops more tender and flavorful.

9. Garnish with lemon wedges and fresh parsley if desired.

10. Serve the baked pork chops hot, with your choice of sides such as mashed potatoes, roasted vegetables, or a fresh salad.

92. Rice Porridge with Chicken

Ingredients:
- 1 cup white rice
- 6 cups chicken broth
- 1 boneless, skinless chicken breast or thigh, thinly sliced or diced
- 1 inch piece of ginger, peeled and thinly sliced
- 2 cloves garlic, minced
- Salt and pepper, to taste
- Optional toppings: sliced green onions, chopped cilantro, fried garlic, fried shallots, soy sauce, sesame oil, chili oil, etc.

Instructions:

1. Rinse the rice under cold water until the water runs clear. This helps remove excess starch and ensures a cleaner broth.

2. In a large pot, combine the rice, chicken broth, sliced ginger, minced garlic, salt, and pepper. Bring the mixture to a boil over medium-high heat.

3. Once boiling, reduce the heat to low and let the porridge simmer, stirring occasionally to prevent sticking, for about 30-40 minutes or until the rice has broken down and the porridge has thickened to your desired consistency.

4. Add the thinly sliced or diced chicken breast or thigh to the porridge. Continue to simmer for another 10-15 minutes, or until the chicken is cooked through.

5. Taste the porridge and adjust the seasoning with more salt and pepper if needed.

6. Serve the chicken rice porridge hot, garnished with your choice of toppings such as sliced green onions, chopped cilantro, fried garlic, fried shallots, soy sauce, sesame oil, chili oil, etc.

7. Enjoy your comforting and nourishing Chicken Rice Porridge!

Feel free to adjust the thickness of the porridge by adding more broth or water if it becomes too thick during cooking.

93. Cottage Cheese Pancakes

Ingredients:
- 1 cup cottage cheese
- 4 large eggs
- 1/4 cup all-purpose flour
- 1 tablespoon sugar (optional, adjust to taste)
- 1 teaspoon vanilla extract
- 1/4 teaspoon salt
- Butter or oil for cooking

Instructions:

1. In a mixing bowl, combine the cottage cheese, eggs, flour, sugar (if using), vanilla extract, and salt. Mix well until smooth.

2. Heat a non-stick skillet or griddle over medium heat. Add a little butter or oil to coat the surface.

3. Pour about 1/4 cup of the pancake batter onto the skillet for each pancake. Use the back of a spoon to spread the batter into a round shape if needed.

4. Cook the pancakes for 2-3 minutes on one side, or until bubbles form on the surface and the edges start to set.

5. Flip the pancakes and cook for another 1-2 minutes on the other side, or until golden brown and cooked through.

6. Transfer the cooked pancakes to a plate and keep warm while you cook the remaining batter.

7. Serve the cottage cheese pancakes hot, topped with your favorite toppings such as fresh fruit, maple syrup, honey, jam, or Greek yogurt.

8. Enjoy your fluffy and flavorful Cottage Cheese Pancakes for a delicious breakfast or brunch!

You can also add a pinch of cinnamon or nutmeg to the batter for extra flavor if desired.

94. Chicken and Rice Pilaf

Ingredients:
- 1 lb boneless, skinless chicken breasts or thighs, cut into bite-sized pieces
- 1 tablespoon olive oil
- 1 onion, finely chopped
- 2 cloves garlic, minced
- 1 cup long-grain rice (such as basmati or jasmine)
- 2 cups chicken broth
- 1/2 teaspoon ground cumin
- 1/2 teaspoon ground coriander
- 1/4 teaspoon ground turmeric
- 1/4 teaspoon paprika
- Salt and pepper, to taste
- 1/4 cup chopped fresh parsley or cilantro, for garnish (optional)
- Lemon wedges, for serving (optional)

Instructions:
1. In a large skillet or sauté pan, heat the olive oil over medium-high heat. Add the chopped onion and cook until softened, about 5 minutes.

2. Add the minced garlic to the skillet and cook for another 1-2 minutes, until fragrant.

3. Add the chicken pieces to the skillet and cook until browned on all sides, about 5-7 minutes.

4. Stir in the rice, ground cumin, ground coriander, ground turmeric, paprika, salt, and pepper. Cook, stirring constantly, for about 1-2 minutes to toast the rice and spices.

5. Pour in the chicken broth and bring the mixture to a boil. Once boiling, reduce the heat to low, cover the skillet, and let it simmer for about 15-20 minutes, or until the rice is tender and the liquid is absorbed.

6. Remove the skillet from the heat and let it sit, covered, for another 5 minutes to allow the flavors to meld together.

7. Fluff the pilaf with a fork and garnish with chopped fresh parsley or cilantro, if desired.

8. Serve the chicken and rice pilaf hot, with lemon wedges on the side for squeezing over the dish if desired.

95. Creamy Broccoli Soup

Ingredients:
- 4 cups broccoli florets (about 1 large head)
- 1 tablespoon olive oil or butter
- 1 onion, chopped
- 2 cloves garlic, minced
- 4 cups vegetable or chicken broth
- 1 cup milk or cream
- Salt and pepper, to taste
- Pinch of nutmeg (optional)
- Grated cheese, for garnish (optional)

Instructions:

1. In a large pot, heat the olive oil or butter over medium heat. Add the chopped onion and cook until softened, about 5 minutes.

2. Add the minced garlic to the pot and cook for another 1-2 minutes, until fragrant.

3. Add the broccoli florets to the pot and cook for about 5 minutes, stirring occasionally, until they start to soften slightly.

4. Pour in the vegetable or chicken broth, making sure the broccoli is submerged. Bring the mixture to a boil.

5. Once boiling, reduce the heat to low and let the soup simmer for about 15-20 minutes, or until the broccoli is tender.

6. Using an immersion blender, blend the soup until smooth and creamy. If you don't have an immersion blender, carefully transfer the soup in batches to a regular blender and blend until smooth. Be cautious with hot liquids.

7. Return the blended soup to the pot (if using a regular blender) and stir in the milk or cream. If you're adding nutmeg, sprinkle it into the soup now.

8. Season the soup with salt and pepper to taste. Adjust the seasoning as needed.

9. Let the soup simmer for another 5 minutes to heat through.

10. Serve the creamy broccoli soup hot, garnished with grated cheese if desired.

96. Turkey and Rice Soup

Ingredients:
- 2 tablespoons olive oil
- 1 onion, chopped
- 2 carrots, diced
- 2 celery stalks, diced
- 2 cloves garlic, minced
- 6 cups turkey or chicken broth
- 2 cups cooked turkey, shredded or diced
- 1 cup cooked rice
- 1 teaspoon dried thyme
- Salt and pepper, to taste
- Chopped fresh parsley, for garnish (optional)

Instructions:

1. In a large pot, heat the olive oil over medium heat. Add the chopped onion, diced carrots, and diced celery. Cook, stirring occasionally, until the vegetables are softened, about 5-7 minutes.

2. Add the minced garlic to the pot and cook for another 1-2 minutes, until fragrant.

3. Pour in the turkey or chicken broth and bring the mixture to a boil.

4. Once boiling, reduce the heat to low and let the soup simmer for about 15-20 minutes, or until the vegetables are tender.

5. Stir in the cooked turkey and cooked rice. Add the dried thyme and season with salt and pepper to taste.

6. Let the soup simmer for another 5-10 minutes to allow the flavors to meld together.

7. Taste the soup and adjust the seasoning as needed.

8. Serve the turkey and rice soup hot, garnished with chopped fresh parsley if desired.

Enjoy your warm and comforting Turkey and Rice Soup!

97. Mashed Butternut Squash

Ingredients:
- 1 medium butternut squash (about 2-3 pounds)
- 2 tablespoons butter
- 2 tablespoons maple syrup (optional)
- Salt and pepper, to taste
- Pinch of ground nutmeg or cinnamon (optional)
- Chopped fresh herbs (such as sage or thyme) for garnish (optional)

Instructions:
1. Preheat your oven to 400°F (200°C).

2. Cut the butternut squash in half lengthwise and scoop out the seeds and fibers from the center using a spoon.

3. Place the squash halves, cut side up, on a baking sheet lined with parchment paper or aluminum foil.

4. Roast the squash in the preheated oven for about 40-50 minutes, or until the flesh is tender when pierced with a fork.

5. Remove the squash from the oven and let it cool slightly.

6. Once cooled, scoop the flesh out of the squash halves and transfer it to a mixing bowl.

7. Add the butter and maple syrup (if using) to the bowl with the squash.

8. Using a potato masher or fork, mash the squash until smooth and creamy. If you prefer a smoother texture, you can also use a hand blender or food processor.

9. Season the mashed butternut squash with salt, pepper, and a pinch of ground nutmeg or cinnamon if desired. Adjust the seasoning to taste.

10. Transfer the mashed butternut squash to a serving dish and garnish with chopped fresh herbs, if desired.

11. Serve the mashed butternut squash hot as a delicious side dish.

Enjoy your flavorful and creamy Mashed Butternut Squash!

98. Chicken and Dumplings

Ingredients:
For the Chicken Stew:
- 1 tablespoon olive oil
- 1 onion, chopped
- 2 carrots, diced
- 2 celery stalks, diced
- 2 cloves garlic, minced
- 4 cups chicken broth
- 2 cups cooked chicken, shredded or diced
- 1 teaspoon dried thyme
- Salt and pepper, to taste
- 1 cup frozen peas (optional)
- Chopped fresh parsley, for garnish (optional)

For the Dumplings:
- 1 cup all-purpose flour
- 2 teaspoons baking powder
- 1/2 teaspoon salt
- 1/2 cup milk
- 2 tablespoons butter, melted

Instructions:
1. In a large pot, heat the olive oil over medium heat. Add the chopped onion, diced carrots, and diced celery. Cook, stirring occasionally, until the vegetables are softened, about 5-7 minutes.

2. Add the minced garlic to the pot and cook for another 1-2 minutes, until fragrant.

3. Pour in the chicken broth and bring the mixture to a boil.

4. Once boiling, reduce the heat to low and let the stew simmer for about 10-15 minutes, allowing the flavors to meld together.

5. Stir in the cooked chicken and dried thyme. Season the stew with salt and pepper to taste.

6. If using frozen peas, add them to the pot and cook for an additional 2-3 minutes, or until heated through.

7. Meanwhile, prepare the dumplings. In a mixing bowl, combine the flour, baking powder, and salt. Stir in the milk and melted butter until a thick batter forms.

8. Drop spoonfuls of the dumpling batter onto the simmering stew. Cover the pot and let the dumplings cook for about 15 minutes, or until they are cooked through and fluffy.

9. Once the dumplings are cooked, remove the pot from the heat.

10. Serve the chicken and dumplings hot, garnished with chopped fresh parsley if desired.

99. Cheese Grits

Ingredients:
- 1 cup stone-ground grits
- 4 cups water or chicken broth
- 1 teaspoon salt
- 1 cup shredded cheddar cheese
- 2 tablespoons butter
- Salt and pepper, to taste

Instructions:

1. In a medium saucepan, bring the water or chicken broth to a boil over high heat.

2. Once boiling, gradually stir in the grits and salt.

3. Reduce the heat to low and let the grits simmer, stirring occasionally, for about 20-25 minutes or until thickened and creamy.

4. Stir in the shredded cheddar cheese and butter until melted and well combined.

5. Season the cheese grits with salt and pepper to taste. Adjust the seasoning as needed.

6. Remove the saucepan from the heat and let the cheese grits sit for a few minutes to thicken further before serving.

7. Serve the cheese grits hot as a delicious side dish or breakfast option.

Enjoy your creamy and flavorful Cheese Grits!

100. Creamed Spinach

Ingredients:
- 1 lb fresh spinach leaves, washed and stems removed
- 2 tablespoons butter
- 2 cloves garlic, minced
- 2 tablespoons all-purpose flour
- 1 cup milk or heavy cream
- 1/4 teaspoon ground nutmeg
- Salt and pepper, to taste
- 1/4 cup grated Parmesan cheese (optional, for extra flavor)

Instructions:

1. Bring a large pot of water to a boil. Add the spinach leaves and blanch for about 1-2 minutes, until wilted. Drain the spinach and rinse under cold water to stop the cooking process. Squeeze out excess water from the spinach and roughly chop it.

2. In a large skillet or sauté pan, melt the butter over medium heat. Add the minced garlic and cook for about 1 minute, until fragrant.

3. Sprinkle the flour over the butter and garlic mixture. Stir well to combine and cook for another 1-2 minutes, until the flour is lightly golden.

4. Gradually pour in the milk or heavy cream, whisking constantly to prevent lumps from forming. Cook, stirring constantly, until the mixture thickens and comes to a simmer, about 3-5 minutes.

5. Stir in the ground nutmeg and season the sauce with salt and pepper to taste.

6. Add the chopped spinach to the sauce and stir to combine. Cook for another 2-3 minutes, until the spinach is heated through and coated in the creamy sauce.

7. If using, sprinkle grated Parmesan cheese over the creamed spinach and stir until melted and well incorporated.

8. Remove the skillet from the heat and transfer the creamed spinach to a serving dish.

9. Serve the creamed spinach hot as a delicious side dish.

Enjoy your creamy and flavorful Creamed Spinach!

101. Baked Cod

Ingredients:
- 4 cod fillets (about 6 ounces each)
- 2 tablespoons olive oil
- 2 cloves garlic, minced
- 1 tablespoon lemon juice
- 1 teaspoon dried parsley
- Salt and pepper, to taste
- Lemon slices, for garnish (optional)
- Chopped fresh parsley, for garnish (optional)

Instructions:
1. Preheat your oven to 400°F (200°C). Lightly grease a baking dish with olive oil or cooking spray.

2. Place the cod fillets in the prepared baking dish in a single layer.

3. In a small bowl, whisk together the olive oil, minced garlic, lemon juice, dried parsley, salt, and pepper.

4. Drizzle the olive oil mixture over the cod fillets, making sure to coat them evenly.

5. If desired, place a lemon slice on top of each cod fillet for extra flavor and presentation.

6. Bake the cod in the preheated oven for about 12-15 minutes, or until the fish is opaque and flakes easily with a fork.

7. Remove the baking dish from the oven and let the cod rest for a few minutes before serving.

8. Garnish the baked cod with chopped fresh parsley if desired.

9. Serve the baked cod hot, accompanied by your favorite side dishes such as roasted vegetables, rice, or salad.

Enjoy your delicious and tender Baked Cod!

102. Soft Tuna Casserole

Ingredients:
- 8 oz (about 225g) egg noodles
- 2 cans (about 10.5 oz each) of canned tuna, drained
- 1 cup frozen peas, thawed
- 1 cup sliced mushrooms
- 1/2 cup chopped onion
- 2 cloves garlic, minced
- 2 tablespoons butter
- 2 tablespoons all-purpose flour
- 2 cups milk
- 1 cup shredded cheddar cheese
- Salt and pepper to taste
- 1/2 cup breadcrumbs (optional)
- Chopped parsley for garnish (optional)

Instructions:

1. Preheat your oven to 350°F (175°C). Grease a baking dish and set aside.

2. Cook the egg noodles according to the package instructions until al dente. Drain and set aside.

3. In a large skillet, melt the butter over medium heat. Add the chopped onion, minced garlic, and sliced mushrooms. Cook until the vegetables are soft and the onions are translucent, about 5-7 minutes.

4. Sprinkle the flour over the vegetables and stir well to combine. Cook for another 2 minutes, stirring constantly.

5. Gradually pour in the milk, stirring constantly to prevent lumps from forming. Cook until the sauce thickens, about 5 minutes.

6. Stir in the shredded cheddar cheese until melted and well combined. Season with salt and pepper to taste.

7. Add the drained tuna and thawed peas to the cheese sauce, stirring gently to combine.

8. Add the cooked egg noodles to the tuna mixture and stir until everything is evenly coated.

9. Transfer the mixture to the prepared baking dish and spread it out evenly. If desired, sprinkle breadcrumbs over the top for added crunch.

10. Bake in the preheated oven for 25-30 minutes, or until the casserole is heated through and bubbly around the edges.

11. Remove from the oven and let it cool for a few minutes before serving. Garnish with chopped parsley if desired. Serve warm and enjoy your comforting soft tuna casserole!

103. Vanilla Rice Pudding

Ingredients:
- 1/2 cup (100g) white rice (long-grain or medium-grain)
- 4 cups (946ml) whole milk
- 1/2 cup (100g) granulated sugar
- 1/4 teaspoon salt
- 1 vanilla bean (or 2 teaspoons vanilla extract)
- Ground cinnamon, for garnish (optional)
- Raisins or dried fruit (optional)

Instructions:

1. Rinse the rice under cold water until the water runs clear. This removes excess starch from the rice.

2. In a medium-sized, heavy-bottomed saucepan, combine the rinsed rice, whole milk, granulated sugar, and salt.

3. If you're using a vanilla bean, split it lengthwise with a sharp knife and scrape out the seeds. Add both the seeds and the vanilla bean pod to the saucepan. If you're using vanilla extract, you'll add it later.

4. Place the saucepan over medium heat and bring the mixture to a gentle simmer, stirring frequently to prevent the rice from sticking to the bottom of the pan.

5. Once the mixture starts simmering, reduce the heat to low and let it cook uncovered, stirring occasionally, for about 25-30 minutes or until the rice is tender and the mixture has thickened to your desired consistency.

6. If you're using vanilla extract instead of a vanilla bean, stir it into the pudding once it has finished cooking.

7. Once the pudding reaches the desired consistency, remove it from the heat. If you prefer a smoother texture, you can remove the vanilla bean pod at this point.

8. Transfer the pudding to serving bowls or glasses. You can serve it warm or chilled, depending on your preference.

9. If desired, sprinkle ground cinnamon over the top of each serving for added flavor and decoration. You can also add raisins or other dried fruit if you like. Enjoy your creamy and comforting vanilla rice pudding!

104. Scrambled Tofu Breakfast Burrito

Ingredients:
- 1 block of firm tofu, drained and pressed
- 1 tablespoon olive oil
- 1/2 onion, diced
- 1 bell pepper, diced
- 2 cloves garlic, minced
- 1 teaspoon ground cumin
- 1/2 teaspoon ground turmeric
- 1/4 teaspoon paprika
- Salt and pepper, to taste
- 1/4 cup nutritional yeast (optional, for extra flavor)
- 1/4 cup chopped fresh cilantro (optional)
- 4 large flour tortillas
- Salsa, avocado slices, shredded cheese, or other toppings of your choice

Instructions:

1. Start by preparing the scrambled tofu. Crumble the pressed tofu into a bowl using your hands or a fork.

2. Heat olive oil in a large skillet over medium heat. Add the diced onion and bell pepper, and sauté until they start to soften, about 3-4 minutes.

3. Add the minced garlic to the skillet and cook for another minute until fragrant.

4. Add the crumbled tofu to the skillet, along with the ground cumin, ground turmeric, paprika, salt, and pepper. Stir well to combine, ensuring that the tofu is evenly coated with the spices.

5. Cook the tofu mixture for about 5-7 minutes, stirring occasionally, until the tofu is heated through and begins to lightly brown.

6. If using, stir in the nutritional yeast for extra flavor and the chopped cilantro for freshness. Adjust seasoning to taste.

7. Warm the flour tortillas in a separate skillet or in the microwave according to package instructions.

8. Divide the scrambled tofu mixture evenly among the warmed tortillas, placing it in the center of each tortilla.

9. Add any additional toppings you like, such as salsa, avocado slices, shredded cheese, or hot sauce.

10. Fold in the sides of each tortilla, then roll it up tightly into a burrito shape. Serve immediately, or wrap the burritos in foil to keep warm until ready to serve. Enjoy your delicious and satisfying Scrambled Tofu Breakfast Burritos!

105. Mashed Parsnips

Ingredients:
- 1 pound (about 450g) parsnips, peeled and chopped into chunks
- 2-3 tablespoons butter or olive oil
- 1/4 cup (60ml) milk or cream (optional)
- Salt and pepper, to taste
- Chopped fresh parsley or chives for garnish (optional)

Instructions:

1. Start by peeling the parsnips and chopping them into evenly sized chunks.

2. Place the parsnip chunks in a large pot and cover them with water. Add a pinch of salt to the water.

3. Bring the water to a boil over medium-high heat, then reduce the heat to medium-low and let the parsnips simmer for about 15-20 minutes, or until they are fork-tender.

4. Once the parsnips are tender, drain them well and return them to the pot.

5. Using a potato masher or fork, mash the parsnips until they reach your desired consistency. If you prefer a smoother texture, you can also use a blender or food processor to puree the parsnips.

6. Stir in the butter or olive oil until it's melted and well incorporated into the mashed parsnips. This will add richness and flavor to the dish.

7. If you like your mashed parsnips creamier, you can stir in some milk or cream at this point. Start with a small amount and add more as needed until you reach your desired consistency.

8. Season the mashed parsnips with salt and pepper to taste. Remember that parsnips have a naturally sweet flavor, so you may not need much seasoning.

9. Transfer the mashed parsnips to a serving dish and garnish with chopped fresh parsley or chives if desired.

10. Serve hot as a delicious side dish alongside your favorite main course.

Enjoy your creamy and flavorful Mashed Parsnips! They make a wonderful alternative to mashed potatoes and are perfect for any occasion.

106. Creamy Asparagus Soup

Ingredients:
- 1 lb (about 450g) fresh asparagus
- 2 tablespoons butter or olive oil
- 1 onion, chopped
- 2 cloves garlic, minced
- 4 cups (946ml) vegetable broth
- 1 medium potato, peeled and diced
- 1/2 cup (120ml) heavy cream (or substitute with coconut cream for a dairy-free option)
- Salt and pepper, to taste
- Lemon juice, to taste (optional)
- Fresh chopped chives or parsley, for garnish (optional)

Instructions:

1. Begin by preparing the asparagus. Wash the asparagus spears and trim off the woody ends. Cut the asparagus into 1-inch pieces, reserving a few spears for garnish if desired.

2. In a large pot or Dutch oven, melt the butter or heat the olive oil over medium heat. Add the chopped onion and sauté until it becomes translucent, about 5 minutes.

3. Add the minced garlic to the pot and sauté for another minute until fragrant.

4. Add the diced potato and asparagus pieces (excluding any reserved for garnish) to the pot. Stir to combine with the onion and garlic.

5. Pour in the vegetable broth, making sure the asparagus and potatoes are submerged. Bring the mixture to a boil, then reduce the heat to medium-low and let it simmer for about 15-20 minutes, or until the vegetables are tender.

6. Once the vegetables are cooked, use an immersion blender to puree the soup until smooth. Alternatively, you can carefully transfer the soup in batches to a blender and blend until smooth, then return it to the pot.

7. Stir in the heavy cream (or coconut cream) until well combined. If the soup is too thick, you can add more broth or water to reach your desired consistency.

8. Season the soup with salt and pepper to taste. If you'd like to add a bright, citrusy flavor, you can also stir in a squeeze of lemon juice.

9. If using, blanch the reserved asparagus spears in boiling water for 2-3 minutes until they are bright green and tender. Remove them from the water and set aside for garnish.

10. Ladle the creamy asparagus soup into bowls. Garnish each bowl with a few reserved asparagus spears and a sprinkle of fresh chopped chives or parsley. Serve hot and enjoy your delicious and comforting Creamy Asparagus Soup!

107. Cheese Tortellini

Ingredients:
- 1 pound (about 450g) cheese tortellini (fresh or frozen)
- Salt, for boiling water
- 2 tablespoons olive oil
- 2 cloves garlic, minced
- 1 can (14.5 oz) diced tomatoes
- 1/2 teaspoon dried basil
- 1/2 teaspoon dried oregano
- Salt and pepper, to taste
- Grated Parmesan cheese, for serving
- Fresh basil leaves, for garnish (optional)

Instructions:

1. Bring a large pot of salted water to a boil. Cook the cheese tortellini according to the package instructions until they are al dente. If using fresh tortellini, they will cook much faster than frozen, typically in just a few minutes. Frozen tortellini may take a bit longer, usually around 8-10 minutes.

2. While the tortellini are cooking, heat the olive oil in a large skillet over medium heat. Add the minced garlic to the skillet and sauté for about 1 minute until fragrant.

3. Stir in the diced tomatoes (with their juices) into the skillet with the garlic. Add the dried basil and oregano, and season with salt and pepper to taste. Allow the mixture to simmer for about 5-7 minutes, stirring occasionally, to let the flavors meld together.

4. Once the tortellini are cooked, drain them well and add them directly to the skillet with the tomato sauce. Toss gently to coat the tortellini evenly with the sauce.

5. Cook for an additional 1-2 minutes, stirring occasionally, until the tortellini are heated through and coated with the sauce.

6. Remove the skillet from the heat. Serve the cheese tortellini hot, garnished with grated Parmesan cheese and fresh basil leaves if desired.

7. Enjoy your delicious and satisfying Cheese Tortellini as a quick and easy weeknight meal!

Feel free to customize this recipe by adding your favorite vegetables, protein, or additional herbs and spices to the tomato sauce for extra flavor. It's a versatile dish that you can make your own!

108. Baked Tilapia

Ingredients:
- 4 tilapia fillets
- 2 tablespoons olive oil
- 2 cloves garlic, minced
- 1 lemon, sliced
- Salt and pepper, to taste
- 1 teaspoon paprika
- 1/2 teaspoon dried thyme
- 1/2 teaspoon dried oregano
- Fresh parsley, chopped, for garnish
- Lemon wedges, for serving

Instructions:

1. Preheat your oven to 400°F (200°C). Grease a baking dish large enough to fit the tilapia fillets in a single layer.

2. Place the tilapia fillets in the prepared baking dish. Drizzle olive oil over the fillets and rub minced garlic onto each fillet.

3. Season the tilapia with salt, pepper, paprika, dried thyme, and dried oregano. Make sure to season both sides of the fillets evenly.

4. Place lemon slices on top of each tilapia fillet.

5. Bake in the preheated oven for 12-15 minutes, or until the fish is opaque and flakes easily with a fork.

6. Once baked, remove the tilapia from the oven and garnish with freshly chopped parsley.

7. Serve the baked tilapia hot with lemon wedges on the side for squeezing over the fish.

8. Enjoy your delicious and flavorful Baked Tilapia as a healthy and satisfying meal!

Feel free to adjust the seasonings and add your favorite herbs and spices to customize the flavor of the tilapia to your liking. You can also add a splash of white wine or a drizzle of melted butter for extra richness, if desired.

109. Chicken Rice Congee

Ingredients:
- 1 cup white rice
- 6 cups chicken broth (or water)
- 1 boneless, skinless chicken breast or thigh, thinly sliced
- 1-inch piece of ginger, thinly sliced
- 2 cloves garlic, minced
- Salt and pepper, to taste
- Optional toppings: chopped green onions, cilantro, fried shallots, sliced ginger, soy sauce, sesame oil

Instructions:

1. Rinse the white rice under cold water until the water runs clear. This helps remove excess starch.

2. In a large pot, combine the rinsed rice, chicken broth (or water), sliced ginger, minced garlic, and a pinch of salt. Bring to a boil over high heat.

3. Once boiling, reduce the heat to low and cover the pot partially with a lid, leaving a small opening to allow steam to escape. Let the congee simmer gently for about 1 to 1.5 hours, stirring occasionally to prevent sticking. The longer you cook, the creamier the congee will become.

4. After the congee has been simmering for about 30 minutes, add the thinly sliced chicken breast or thigh to the pot. Continue to simmer until the chicken is cooked through and the congee reaches your desired consistency. If the congee becomes too thick, you can add more broth or water to thin it out.

5. Season the congee with salt and pepper to taste.

6. Ladle the chicken rice congee into bowls. Serve hot with your choice of toppings such as chopped green onions, cilantro, fried shallots, sliced ginger, soy sauce, or sesame oil.

7. Enjoy your warm and comforting Chicken Rice Congee!

Feel free to adjust the seasoning and thickness of the congee according to your taste preferences. It's a versatile dish that you can customize with your favorite ingredients and toppings.

110. Creamy Vegetable Soup

Ingredients:
- 2 tablespoons butter or olive oil
- 1 onion, diced
- 2 cloves garlic, minced
- 2 carrots, peeled and diced
- 2 celery stalks, diced
- 1 large potato, peeled and diced
- 4 cups (946ml) vegetable broth
- 2 cups (480ml) milk or cream
- 2 cups mixed vegetables (such as broccoli florets, cauliflower florets, peas, corn, etc.)
- 1/2 teaspoon dried thyme
- Salt and pepper, to taste
- Chopped fresh parsley or chives, for garnish (optional)

Instructions:

1. In a large pot or Dutch oven, melt the butter over medium heat. Add the diced onion and sauté until it becomes translucent, about 5 minutes.

2. Add the minced garlic to the pot and cook for another minute until fragrant.

3. Add the diced carrots, celery, and potato to the pot. Stir to combine with the onion and garlic.

4. Pour in the vegetable broth and bring the mixture to a boil. Once boiling, reduce the heat to medium-low and let it simmer for about 10-15 minutes, or until the vegetables are tender.

5. Once the vegetables are cooked, use an immersion blender to puree the soup until smooth. Alternatively, you can carefully transfer the soup in batches to a blender and blend until smooth, then return it to the pot.

6. Stir in the milk or cream until well combined.

7. Add the mixed vegetables and dried thyme to the pot. Let the soup simmer for another 5-10 minutes, or until the vegetables are heated through.

8. Season the soup with salt and pepper to taste.

9. Ladle the creamy vegetable soup into bowls. Garnish each bowl with chopped fresh parsley or chives if desired. Serve hot and enjoy your comforting and creamy Vegetable Soup!

Feel free to customize this recipe by using your favorite vegetables or adding herbs and spices according to your taste preferences. It's a versatile and nutritious dish that's perfect for any occasion.

111. Turkey and Mashed Potato Casserole

Ingredients:
- 1 cup shredded cheddar cheese
- 1/2 cup milk
- 2 tablespoons butter
- Salt and pepper, to taste
- Optional toppings: chopped fresh parsley, breadcrumbs
- 2 cups cooked turkey, shredded or diced
- 4 cups mashed potatoes (about 2 lbs potatoes)
- 1 cup frozen mixed vegetables (such as peas, carrots, corn)

Instructions:

1. Preheat your oven to 375°F (190°C). Grease a 9x13 inch baking dish and set aside.

2. In a large mixing bowl, combine the cooked turkey, mashed potatoes, frozen mixed vegetables, and shredded cheddar cheese. Season with salt and pepper to taste. Mix well to combine.

3. Transfer the turkey and mashed potato mixture to the prepared baking dish, spreading it out evenly.

4. In a small saucepan, heat the milk and butter over medium heat until the butter is melted and the mixture is warm.

5. Pour the warm milk and butter mixture evenly over the top of the casserole.

6. If desired, sprinkle breadcrumbs over the top of the casserole for added crunch.

7. Cover the baking dish with aluminum foil and bake in the preheated oven for 20-25 minutes, or until the casserole is heated through and bubbly around the edges.

8. Remove the foil and continue baking for an additional 5-10 minutes, or until the top is golden brown and crispy.

9. Once baked, remove the casserole from the oven and let it cool for a few minutes before serving.

10. Garnish with chopped fresh parsley if desired. Serve warm and enjoy your delicious Turkey and Mashed Potato Casserole!

This casserole is a great way to use up leftover turkey from holiday meals, and it's a comforting and hearty dish that the whole family will love. Feel free to customize it with your favorite seasonings or additional ingredients!

As we reach the conclusion of **"110+ Low-Fiber Recipes for Diverticulitis: Gentle and Delicious Meals,"** we hope that this collection has provided you with a variety of enjoyable and soothing meal options tailored to your specific dietary needs. Managing diverticulitis can be a complex journey, but with the right knowledge and resources, it is possible to maintain a fulfilling and nutritious diet.

The recipes within these pages have been carefully designed to offer relief and comfort, ensuring that you can enjoy delicious meals without exacerbating your condition. From breakfasts that gently wake up your digestive system to dinners that provide satisfaction without strain, each dish has been crafted with your health and enjoyment in mind.

Throughout this book, we have emphasized the importance of understanding your dietary needs and making informed choices. The insights and tips provided aim to empower you to take control of your health through mindful eating. By adhering to a low-fiber diet during flare-ups and incorporating these gentle recipes into your routine, you can help manage symptoms and promote healing.

We hope that the variety of recipes has inspired you to experiment in the kitchen and find joy in cooking. Whether you are preparing meals for yourself or for loved ones, the ease and flavor of these dishes will make mealtime a pleasurable and stress-free experience.

In addition to the recipes, the practical advice on meal planning, ingredient selection, and cooking techniques is designed to support you in making consistent, healthful choices. We encourage you to continue exploring and adapting these recipes to suit your preferences and nutritional needs, knowing that you have a solid foundation to build upon.

"110+ Low-Fiber Recipes for Diverticulitis" is not just a cookbook but a companion in your journey towards better health. By incorporating these meals into your diet, you can enjoy the dual benefits of delicious food and symptom management, leading to a more balanced and enjoyable lifestyle.

Thank you for allowing us to be a part of your culinary and health journey. May the recipes and knowledge shared here bring you comfort, nourishment, and satisfaction. Here's to your continued health and the many gentle, delicious meals that await you.

Bon appétit and best wishes for a healthy, happy future!